Johnny Come Lately

JOHNNY COME LATELY

A Short History of the Condom

Jeannette Parisot

Translated and enlarged by Bill McCann
New material and revisions by Geraldine Rudge
Illustrations by Bill Piggins

JOURNEYMAN

Originally published by Buntbuch Verlag 1985 as *Dein Kondom — das unbekannte Wesen*, this English translation has been completely revised, and is first published in Great Britain by the Journeyman Press, March 1987, as *Johnny Come Lately: A Short History of the Condom*.

The Journeyman Press Ltd, 97 Ferme Park Road, London N8 9SA

ISBN 1 85172 000 6 (new series)

Cover illustration by Bill Piggins

First edition 1987

87 88 89 90 91 92 93   10 9 8 7 6 5 4 3 2 1

Typeset by SMC Typesetting and printed by Robert Hartnoll (1985) Ltd, Bodmin

Acknowledgements

So many people helped us with the research for this book we cannot mention them all, but our special thanks must be given to Helga Stochow of the University of Hamburg, Bill McCann of the University of Southampton and Geraldine Rudge for the valuable information they provided.

Journeyman would also like to thank *City Limits, Time Out, New Statesman* and *Forum* for the editorial support they gave its survey in 1986, Michael Conitzer of Jiffi Ltd, Patrick Moylett of Fredrick Trading Company and Clive Gore of Aegis Ltd for the condoms they provided for testing, and last but not least, the many survey participants who struggled to complete the questionnaire.

In addition, Journeyman would also like to record its appreciation for the co-operation it received from the following: Stephanie Ratkai of the Dudley Castle Archaeological Project; Mr Calnan of the Leather Conservation Centre, Northampton; Lesley Hall of the Wellcome Institute Library; Rita Ward and Philip Meredith of the IPPF; Philip Kestelman; Charlotte Owen and Kaye Wellings of the FPA; Arlette Campbell-White of the HEC; the Department of Medieval and Later Antiquities at the British Museum; Liz and Joe Page; Joy Chamberlin; Roger Wood; and many others who have warmly welcomed the publication of this book.

Illustrations have been reproduced with the kind permission of the following sources: Wellcome Institute Library, London, 15, 31. George Allen & Unwin Ltd: *Birth Control Methods* by Norman Haire (1941), 2, 14. Dudley Castle Archaeological Project, 3, 4. Library of Congress, Washington DC, 5. British Library, 12. Trustees of the British Museum, 6, 9, 10, 11. GGK Publicity Agency, 26. Stuart Franklin, Magnum Photos, Paris, 16, 17. International Planned Parenthood Federation, 20, 21, 22, 23, 24, 29. Fredrick Trading Company, London, 25. SOMARC, New York, 28. Bill McCann, 32. Harper & Row, Publishers: *Vaginal Contraception: New Developments* edited by G. I. Zatuchni (1979), 27.

Quotations have been made with the kind permission of the following copyright owners: Secker & Warburg Ltd: Malcolm Bradbury *Eating People is Wrong*; Tom Sharpe *Wilt, The Throwback* and *Porterhouse Blue*; David Lodge *Ginger You're Barmy*. The Estate of the late Sonia Brownell Orwell and Secker & Warburg Ltd: George Orwell *Keep the Aspidistra Flying*. Chatto &

Windus Ltd: Aldous Huxley *Brave New World*: Josef Skvorecky *The Engineer of Human Souls*; Lisa Alther *Kinflicks*. Jonathan Cape Ltd: Philip Roth *Portnoy's Complaint*; John Irving *Cider House Rules*; Michael Joseph Ltd: Wendy Perriam *Born of Woman* and *The Stillness, the Dancing*; Stan Barstow *A Kind of Loving*. Brian W. Aldiss: *Hand-Reared Boy* and *A Soldier Erect* (published by Transworld). J P Donleavy: *The Ginger Man* (published by Penguin Books).

The following were referred to during additional research: Wm E Kruck *Looking for Dr Condom* (University of North Carolina, 1981); S Green *The Curious History of Contraception* (London, 1971); B E Finch and H Green *Contraception Through the Ages* (London, 1963); *The History of Contraceptives* (8th Conference of IPPF, Santiago, Chile, 1967); *Social Marketing Update* (Vol 6, No 2, Summer, New York, 1986); G Seneviratne 'A rebirth of faith in the condom' *People News and Features* (IPPF, London, 1986); N E Himes *The Medical History of Contraception* (New York, 1963); P Fryer *The Birth Controllers* (London, 1965).

This book is dedicated to the man who, in November 1984, wrote about a new contraceptive in the French paper *La Libération*, and was quoted in several European dailies. This new contraceptive had recently been introduced into France. The writer had no interest in its side-effects on women, but was worried about something entirely different: it would 'more than ever exclude men from contraception'. He also explained that 'currently one out of two French women do not use a contraceptive'. Unfortunately he forgot to enlighten us about French men's contraceptive habits. But if they suffer so much being excluded from contraception . . . well, help is here! They can use a condom . . . so this book is also dedicated to them.

LRC Products Ltd

North Circular Road London E4 8QA
Telephone: 01-527 2377
Telex: 21644
Facsimile: 015310060
Telegrams: Lonrubmanf London Telex

A member of the London International Group plc

RRT/SS   15th July 1986

Mr P. Sinclair,
Journeyman Press Ltd.,
97, Ferne Park Road,
Crouch End,
LONDON N8 9JA.

Dear Mr Sinclair,

This is to inform you that the Company has decided that it will not
participate in the Journeyman Press "Condom Survey", or give
permission for our Registered Trade Mark Durex, or other registered
Durex Sheath brand names to be mentioned or used in any way in this
Survey or any related publication connected with the Survey.

Yours sincerely,
LRC PRODUCTS LTD

R. Ross-Turner

A Condomological Preface

According to Dorland's *Medical Dictionary*, a condom is: 'latin *condus*, a receptacle; according to some authorities a corruption of Condon, the inventor. A sheath or cover for the penis, worn during coitus to prevent impregnation or infection'. If by mistake you consult your atlas, you will also find that Condom is a town in France, but we will explain the significance of that later on.

This book is entirely devoted to the condom, also known as a French Letter (if you're English), Capote Anglaise (if you're French), Dibber (if you're a Yuppie) or Port Said Garter (if you're a historian).

For our purposes we have opted to use the word 'condom' to describe the contraceptive, and 'penis' to describe the part of the anatomy it is made-to-measure for. Occasionally, though, we have reverted to French Letter, sheath or even rubber – if only to relieve you from unnecessary repetition!

However, as you will see from the letter from LRC Products Ltd reproduced opposite, we have been forbidden to mention the word '███████'. Doubtless, had we done so, a legal threat might have prevented you, dear Reader, from purchasing this book. So, to safeguard LRC's legal right of sole use of their Registered Trade Mark, we have scrupulously avoided making any mention of '███████' throughout our text. But, if you should find one that we have inadvertently missed, please close your eyes and cross it through before you read it – otherwise great harm could be done to the publisher, distributor, printer, bookseller and author! Of course, it is somewhat ironic that just as the condom is likely to become 'normalised', in the words of an LRC director, their refusal to help during the preparation of the only history of the condom in the English language has resulted in it being published without referring to their brands by name. Somewhat shortsighted, we should have said.

Contents

List of Illustrations

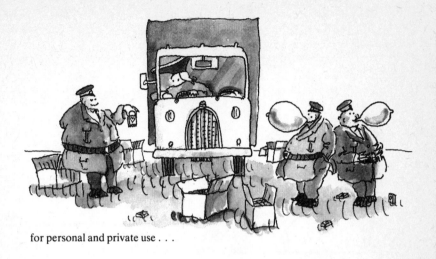

for personal and private use . . .

The Curious and Wonderful
History of the Condom

If we ask ourselves 'What do we know about the history of the condom?', then, like Shakespeare (whose only reference to the condom appears to have been to call it a 'Venus glove'), we have to answer 'Little more than a little'.

Possibly the earliest example of its use is depicted in a cave painting at Les Combarelles in the Department of Dordogne, France, dated at between 15,000 BC and 10,000 BC. There a man is shown in the act, apparently sheathed.

More than 3000 years ago the Egyptians were wearing fine linen sheaths (with very little else), but mostly for decoration, doubling as a coloured badge of rank and a defence against insects and tropical diseases. Even today, Dani tribesmen of the Indonesian valley town of Wamena can still be seen wearing only a *koteka* (penis-gourd). Doubtless this sight will soon vanish as they are forced to join twentieth-century 'civilisation'. Another primitive tribe, the Djukas in South America, were known to have used a seed pod. More a female condom, one end was cut off and then placed closed end first, high in the woman's vagina. Hardly comfortable, but no less than the tortoiseshell or horn *kabutogata* (hard helmets) used by the Japanese before the invention of rubber condoms (but they also made a thin leather sheath, known as a *kawagata* or *kyotai*, so it wasn't always quite so painful).

Some 2000 years ago the Chinese were using oiled silk paper,

1

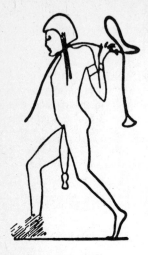

1. A sketch of an ancient Egyptian non-contraceptive sheath, 1350 BC–1200 BC. As much a badge of rank as a likely defence against flies.

befitting a society which invented paper. But it was the Greeks and Romans who can claim the first distinction of using an animal membrane, and in particular King Minos of Crete. That's right, the one who had the labyrinth built to house the Minotaur. He had the socially unacceptable habit of ejaculating snakes and scorpions, with fatal results for his unfortunate partners. It was possibly his palace inventor Daedalus who came up with the idea of inserting a goat's bladder into the young woman who was to be honoured in this way, so that Minos could shoot his serpentine load without harming her. However, the question arises whether this can really be considered a remote ancestor of the condom – maybe it was more a form of diaphragm? There is also the likelihood that Roman soldiers, in the true tradition of all 'civilising' armies, used the tough connecting tissue sheaths of long muscles, cut from the bodies of their slain enemies.

But, like all our predecessors, it seems we must return to the scientific writers of antiquity in our search for the primal condom. Aristotle is mentioned as an early user (though without any evidence having been found in his writings – so far), and also Pliny, who usually finds a place in these discussions.

The Case of Pliny

The French Letter question, when asked about Pliny, produces the answer, 'Nothing, not a sausage'. Classical dictionaries are no help at all. The sort of thing you get is: 'Pliny (1) The Elder (Gaius P Secundus), Roman author and scientific writer, b Comum AD

23/24, d 79 in the eruption of Vesuvius. As an officer travelled widely in the Roman Empire. Apart from a few fragments, most of the Pliny's grammatical, historical, rhetorical, military and biographical writings have been lost.'

What evidence does this provide of Pliny's contraceptive practices? As a well-travelled author, he would probably always have had a French (or Gaulish?) Letter tucked away in the folds of his toga: prophylactic provision has always played a large role in military life, and the last war gives us several examples. Even in Nazi Germany, when contraception was in bad odour and a decree directly from Himmler forbade the sale of condoms in public places, an exception was made for the members of the Wehrmacht. They were not only allowed to use them, they had to, so that their strength and will to fight wouldn't be sapped by a carelessly contracted infection.

After the publication of the German edition of this book, an old gentleman wrote in to tell of his experiences in the army in the thirties. The soldiers were forbidden to leave barracks without a supply of condoms, but although they could be presented for inspection on the way out, it was impossible to check that they were actually used; so, to make sure they obeyed orders, any soldier who caught VD was severely punished – in addition to the agony of its treatment in those pre-penicillin days. John Masters' autobiography also mentions wartime condom usage, though of a totally different kind: since our lads were obviously too virtuous to have any other use for them, they used them in the rivers and jungles of the Far East to keep their weapons and possessions dry (a practice that still obtains in the Australian army, see 'Condom Curiosities'). The Second World War naval rating was no less ingenious when it came to finding an alternative use. One ex-sailor we spoke to kept a handy survival pack in a condom: a bar of chocolate, a packet of fags and a box of matches – just in case the boat sank. And when objections have been made to the issue of condoms to the military, the reasons have not always been of the most moral: Norwegian soldiers sent to Germany in 1945 were prudently issued with French Letters. There was a storm of public protest. Why? Not because they thought that the Norwegian soldiery was too moral to screw around abroad, but because they were convinced that no true Norwegian would sink so low as to get involved with a German. Those who did deserved their punishment.

Fertile and fascinating though such considerations may be, they don't get us any further with Pliny. We can only assume that he didn't travel the Roman Imperium unprotected. His nephew Pliny (the Younger) doesn't help much either. His letters, particularly the one about the eruption of Vesuvius, have been used as instruments of torture in schools for centuries, but the school editions don't say a word about condoms. Perhaps sentences like 'amici firmi eligendi sunt, cuius generis est magna penuria' (you must choose *durable* friends, there is a great dearth of that kind) can be interpreted as a complaint about the poor quality of condoms at the time. None of this, however, helps to fill the gaps in the riddle of the condom.

Why were all the early researchers so obsessed with the idea of Greek and Roman condoms? They were probably under pressure to make the subject respectable. The basic works were written at the beginning of this century, by doctors who were fighting against social prejudice and legal obstacles to make contraception generally available. Proof that they could call on examples from the Glory that was Greece (or Rome) must have worked in their favour. 'Even Aristotle, you say? . . . Well, the Ancient Greeks . . . the cradle of democracy . . . Philosophy, the Parthenon, the language . . . and Homer.' The Member of Parliament (Congress . . .) becomes enthusiastic, and – carried away in a classical frenzy – votes for a bill to allow the sale of condoms to responsible married couples.

The only problem is that these early researchers never tell us what the Great Minds of Antiquity actually wrote. And where they wrote it is also a mystery. After all, who these days knows enough Greek or Latin to plough through the complete works of these people in the hope of coming across the relevant passages? In the end, the evidence (if there is any) remains as safely hidden in those dusty tomes as Pliny's collection of French Letters does under the ashes of Pompeii. But not all may be lost: a certain couple were caught in the act during those last days of Pompeii, and have remained so to this day. It will be a brave condomologist who can discover if they were using one!

The Gloom of the Middle Ages

At the end of the Golden Age of Classical Antiquity Rome declined and fell, and Europe saw the dawn of the Dark Ages (a period in history, about which even less is known). Then came the Crusades, the Black Death and the persecution of witches – this last being the reason why we know nothing about medieval condoms. The women who were said to be witches were accused again and again of having carried out abortions (mortal sin) and prevented conception through the use of contraceptive devices and potions (a thousand times worse than abortion). That contraception should be worse than abortion seems absurd, but it is completely reasonable seen in the light of scholastic logic. In the case of abortion, a soul is already in existence (though the stage of pregnancy at which the soul enters the foetus is, like the number of angels that can balance on the point of a needle, a subject of controversy), and can praise the Lord for all eternity in the limbo to which unbaptised souls are sent. If conception is prevented, God gets nothing at all, not even the tiniest bit of unbaptised soul. Hence the saint and philosopher Thomas Aquinas considers the woman who prevents conception to be worse than a murderer.

No wonder, then, that in such a moral and intellectual climate no brave soul reached for his pen to compose a lay in praise of condoms. At least, not in the Christian West – and so far, very little is known about the non-Christian Orient.

The Comeback of the French Letter

While so-called witches were merrily being exterminated (the last one was burnt as late as 1894, by the way, in Ireland, where French Letters were themselves illegal until 1980, and only became available off prescription in 1985; in both cases, the forces of progress were a bit slower than elsewhere), condoms were heading for a resurgence in the sixteenth century. This was because men, who until very shortly before had considered contraception to be worse than murder, suddenly began to feel the effects of this philosophy on themselves – in a very intimate way. Syphilis was reaching epidemic proportions, especially amongst the upper classes, so the doctors began to look for a solution.

In 1564, in a book published two years after his death, the Italian doctor Gabriello Falloppio (known in Britain for the discovery of the tubes which bear his name) described linen sheaths soaked in herbal brews and inorganic salts, which were intended to prevent infection. Hercules Saxonia also described a similar linen cover in 1597, attributing it to Fallopius. There were two types:

1. A larger sheath to be drawn over the whole penis, like our own French Letters.
2. Smaller sheaths, which were meant to be inserted beneath the foreskin. Unfortunately, there are no illustrations of this mysterious device, and even his instructions leave us none the wiser:

> As often as a man has intercourse, he should (if possible) wash the genitals, or wipe them with a cloth; afterwards he should use a small linen cloth made to fit the *glans*, and draw the prepuce over the *glans*; if he can do so, it is well to moisten it with saliva or with a lotion; however, it does not matter. If you fear lest caries (syphilis) be produced in the canal, take the sheath of this linen cloth and place it in the canal; I tried the experiment on eleven hundred men, and I call immortal God to witness that not one of them was infected.

These Fallopian linen condoms never really caught on – and in the case of the second sort it's easy to see why – so the manufacturers turned to the appendix of the sheep, lamb, calf and goat for their raw material, as you will shortly learn. It is also said that fish bladders were used as well, but on this the authorities disagree.

Some say that it is a very fishy matter which ought to be consigned to the realms of fantasy, and maintain that there is no evidence that anyone ever used a fish bladder as a French Letter. The other side admittedly fails to produce any concrete evidence, but they do produce concrete descriptions. According to them, these strange objects could only be made out of the inner skin of the swim-bladder air-bladder of the sturgeon and the catfish – and they are supposed to have made this up out of their own heads!

Of course they didn't. In Germany on the 11th of October 1910 a 'device for holding fish-bladder condoms in place' was patented, by Patent No 232 797m Class 90d Group 15 of the Imperial Patent Office to be exact. The inventor was a certain Willibald Schaar-schmidt of Leipzig. Why should this latter-day Daedalus have gone to all this trouble, if the fish-bladder condom did not exist? The device for holding them on existed in several variants. This was the basic model:

> 'Device for holding fish-bladder condoms in place, characterised in that, in order to prevent the fish bladder becoming detached in use and to provide a method of handling the same, it comprises a removable, rigid rim at the open end, consisting of two concentric rings which clamp the edge of the condom between them.'

That was the simple model – for more demanding connoisseurs there were the following luxury models:

1. Sprung and fixed elements on the outer ring served to hold the inner ring, which was inserted into it, in place.
2. One of the two rings was rigid, the other was sprung.
3. The outer ring was coated with soft rubber.
4. The rings could be inserted into one another and locked with a twisting movement like a bayonet.

Variant 4 represents without any doubt the highpoint of all possible developments in devices for the attachment of fish-bladder con-doms. The fish which provided these bladders in the good old days are, by the way, nearly extinct in Europe, and certainly in Ger-many; while other fish whose bladders could not be used in con-doms, such as trout and carp, are flourishing. Doesn't that give pause for thought? So, in the interests of condomology, our diligent researches have finally uncovered what may be the only surviving

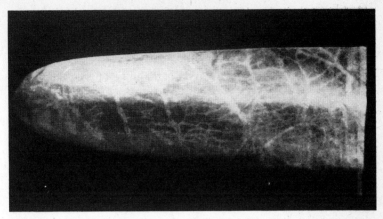

2. A rare photograph of a fish-bladder condom. Made from the air-bladder (not the other sort) of the sturgeon or cat-fish.

photograph of a fish condom, solving one of life's last great mysteries. As you will see, it certainly needs a device to hold it on, and had there been a greater supply of sturgeons and catfish, Willibald Schaarschmidt would doubtless have become a household name.

Still, he was not the only inventor of genius in the latter days of the German Empire. Hot on his heels came Eduard Nitardy of Berlin, who on the 30th of January 1912 patented a 'device for the artificial erection of the penis'. This consisted of 'a hollow body to be placed over the penis, characterised in that the cylindrical hollow body, fitted for that purpose with a suspensory, has an elastic double lining whose interior can be inflated by means of an air-tube fitted with a stopper in such a way that the inner lining encloses the member with the appropriate pressure.' Obviously the only purpose of this device was to allow even more men to make use of Schaarschmidt's excellent device – which takes us back to our proper concern after this short deviation.

One advantage of early condoms was that they could be used several times, but the disadvantage was that they did not stretch. Very few men will have had the cash (or the nerve) to have condoms tailor-made (though there is a rumour that the poet Heinrich Heine had them made of blue silk), and even off the peg they weren't cheap. This tends to suggest that their use was not very widespread.

Gossamer against Danger

The invention of the sheath made of sheep-gut is normally ascribed

to a Dr Condom, Condon, Conton, Controm or something similar,
even though he probably never existed, which is why people have
trouble spelling his name. Condom, so the legend goes, was physician to King Charles II, who like all the Stuarts enjoyed his
pleasures and begat a large number of illegitimate offspring. Dr C.
is said to have invented his device to prevent the throne being
inundated with claimants. This is hardly convincing: in the first
place, the illegitimate children already existed; and secondly, there
were such clear laws of succession that even Henry VIII, who was
just as active, failed to circumvent them – and Henry, holder of the
world record for legal uxoricide, tried every way he could. Anyway,
the stories usually then tell how Charles was so delighted that he
knighted the gallant doctor – who had to change his name as a result
of being connected with such a disgraceful device, which may explain why he has been so difficult to trace.

It was also suggested that he was a Colonel during Charles' reign.
This was based on a note in the 1741 edition of *A Panegyrick upon
Cundum*, written as early as 1723 by Rev White Kennet, the son of
the Bishop of Peterborough. Later editions were published under
the title *Allusion to the Splendid Shilling*. The same note was
repeated in a poem called *The Machine: or, Love's Preservative*
(anonymous) in 1744, with the additional comment that it had
become indecent to mention his name, according to *Tatler*.

As an interesting diversion, what follows is a list of the many
attempts by researchers and others to find out who invented the
condom:

A CONDOM CHRONOLOGY

1705 Edinburgh: Duke of Argyll takes a 'Quondam' north when he enters
      the Scottish Parliament.

1706 Edinburgh: 'Condum' first mentioned in a poem by Lord Belhaven.

1708 London: 'Condon' said to be named after inventor in *Almonds for
      Parrots*.

1709 London: *Tatler* refers to the inventor and his 'Engine', but gives no
      name.

1717 London: Dr Daniel Turner says 'Condum' is the best preservative.

1742 London: Turner says inventor was Dr C____n.

1728 London: In *Allusion to the Splendid Shilling* inventor said to be a
      Colonel.

1738 Paris: Astruc writes that English use skins called 'Condums'.

1773 Paris: Bauchaumont's memoirs refer to 'le Condon'.

1785 London: Inventor was a Col. Cundom according to Grose's slang
      dictionary.

1788 Gottingen: Girtanner says invention named after Condom, its inventor.

1790–97 Paris: Casanova said English invented it.

1795 Paris: Marquis de Sade mentioned it.

1798 Paris: Swediaur claimed Dr Condom changed his name to avoid public scorn.

1847 Vienna: Hyrtl says inventor was a Restoration cavalier called Gondom.

1872 Vienna: Prokosch says inventor was Dr Conton, a Restoration physician.

1888 Oxford: Murray of *N.E.D.* says condom derived from 'Quondam'.

1901 Paris: Cabanès states invention and inventor were from eighteenth-century London.

1904 Hildesheim: Ferdy suggests condom is named after French town.

1905 Paris: Ferdy suggests condom is derived from latin *condus*.

1911 Berlin: Richter proposes that condom is based on the Persian *kondü* or *kendü*, animal intestines used to store grain.

1928 Vienna: *Bilder-Lexicon* suggests name is based on latin *condere gladium*.

1940 Westport: Bernstein proposes Cundum was an English army officer.

1972 Chicago: *Playboy* suggests it is based on 'conundrum'.

1986 London: Journeyman* suggests inventor was an army physician called Quondam.

---

*Journeyman, during painstaking editorial verification of this text, and following a tradition set by the 1728 publisher of *A Panegyric upon Cundum*, has concluded that the inventor was a Royalist army physician called Colonel Quondam, based in the West Midlands. Research connected with the discovery of five condom fragments at Dudley Castle confirm that a Colonel Quondam (related to a previous owner of the castle) and several Cavalier officers were in a desperate situation during a siege of the castle by Cromwell's New Model Army in 1645. Faced with the quandary (a word derived from the Colonel's family name during the previous century, cf *O.E.D.*) of starvation or death at the hands of their enemies, they made an ingenious attempt at escape by disguising themselves as Roundheads. Unfortunately they were unsuccessful – the castle was stormed and after a final battle the Cavaliers suffered a terrible fate (a medieval torture – hacking away skin with a blunt knife). Their tattered disguises were thrown into the garderobe (lavatory) to be discovered almost 350 years later. Fortunately Colonel Quondam survived this ordeal, and to avoid being identified with this defeat, retired from the Army and changed his name to Dr Cundum, which of course is the reason why later scholars have been unable to trace his ancestry. To the end of his life, though, he continued to make copies of the 'disguises' which had been so ineffective in battle. It was not, it seems, until Mrs Philips started commercial production at the turn of the century that 'condums' became popular, more as a barrier against syphilis than a disguise (although in the twentieth century efforts have been made to reintroduce them in this form, with little success).

Other authorities claim that Dr C. lived in the middle of the nineteenth century, and cast doubt on the idea that he invented anything at all. If this is true, then there is no reason why he should be remembered anyway. There is a French legend that an English Dr Condom initiated his French colleague Cullerier into the mysteries of the sheath. This so excited the French Dr C. that he set off hotfoot for France to spread the good news among his long-suffering compatriots. In gratitude they erected a monument to him in the Pere Lachaise cemetery, with the inscription 'Son nom rappelle ses vertus' (His name reminds us of his virtues). But, as is often the case, the name is forgotten, the invention lingers on. Still, most great inventors have been anonymous – we all know who invented the Rolls Royce, but who knows who invented the wheel?

The recent discovery of five animal-gut condom fragments at Dudley Castle in the West Midlands provides us with the earliest surviving examples yet, and somewhat undermines the truth behind the legend that they were invented by Dr C. over a quarter of a century later.

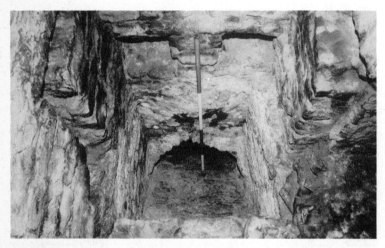

3. Interior of the ground-floor garderobe, or lavatory, in the keep at Dudley Castle, similar to the chute in which five condom fragments were found. The garderobe has been filled with masonry since 1647, making it impossible for anything found lower to be of a later date.

Archaeologists working in the castle's keep found what was left of the condoms in the garderobe, or lavatory, last used by Royalist officers during the English Revolution in the 1640s. Fortunately the fragments had been preserved in a silty layer which prevented them from decomposing, but it was only when a conservator's sharp eye

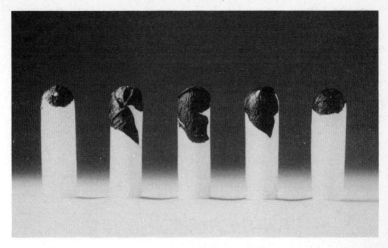

4. The five condom fragments found at Dudley Castle, photographed whilst drying out on 'extraction thimbles'. Only luck prevented them from being overlooked: the archaeologists working at the castle nearly mistook them for leaves, and it was only by chance that the conservator guessed what they were.

noticed how wondrous close fitting they were when placed on the round-ended paper 'extraction thimbles', used as formes during the drying-out process, that it was suspected they were ancient members of the condom family. And since they had been found in the lavatory . . . well, little seems to have changed in 340 years!

By 1666 it seems that they were readily available in London. A witness before the first English Birthrate Commission testified that condoms were in use there at the time of the Great Fire. But whether they were made from animal membrane or linen, we have no information. Certainly linen condoms were known in Paris in 1655. A play that year, called 'L'Escole des filles', possibly by Michel Millot, refers to the use by a man of 'a small cloth' (un petit linge). Even more significant is the context in which it was to be used: Susanne tells her cousine Fanchon that to avoid pregnancy, precautions must be taken. To our knowledge, this is the earliest reference to the use of a condom as a contraceptive device.

In Britain, animal-gut condoms had been steadily increasing in popularity, most probably because the raw material was always at hand as waste from the slaughter-houses. By the turn of the century a certain Mrs Philips was already, in her own words, 'in the business of making and selling machines, commonly called implements of safety, which serves the health of her customers', and in a play attributed to William Burnaby, it is suggested that a condom shop already existed in 1701.

But the actual word condom first appears in 1706, mentioned in a poem called *A Scots Answer to a British Vision* by John Hamilton, 2nd Baron of Belhaven, in which he rhymes 'condum' with John Campbell's (2nd Duke of Argylle) reference to having brought a 'Quondam' north to Scotland the year before:

> Then *Sirenge* and *Condum*
> Come both in Request.
> While virtuous *Quondam*
> Is treated in Jest

More forthcoming is *Almonds for Parrots* (anonymous), published in 1708, which quite definitely assumes that the name is that of the inventor:

> O matchless *Condom*! thou'st secur'd thy Fame
> To last as long as *Condom* is a Name.
> Such mighty things are by thy Influence done,
> Thou ha'st the foremost of this Age out-run.
> *Vulcan* himself has been out-script by thee,
> Thou patron of the *Paphian* Deity.
> For *Mars*'s Heroes, shining Arms he made;
> But thou for *Venus*, takes up *Vulcan*'s Trade.
> Superior much, thou do'st the God out-shine.
> *Achilles* Armour cannot match with thine.
> Thine makes the Knight invulnerable still;
> (. . .)
> *Condon* has quench'd the heat of *Venus*'s Fire,
> And yet preserv'd the Flame of *Love*'s Desire.

Here already we find the use of the term *armour*, and a foreshadowing of later developments in rubber technology in the mention of Vulcan. In view of the scholastic arguments against contraception, it's amusing that this poem assumes that Dr C.'s invention shows the workings of divine providence:

> O *Condon*! bless'd must be thy teeming Brain
> That proves at lenghth [sic], *Nature* made nought in vain
> But such capacious Heads as thine, can find
> For what they were at first by her design'd.
> Long had the Paeans of the Age, who shine
> In Arts, and boast themselves of Race divine;
> Long had these *Aesculapian* Heroes vex'd
> Their leisure Thoughts, and long their Minds perplex'd,
> To search the Cause why *Nature* had assign'd
> To Men and Brutes, a *Gut* the Learn'd call *Blind*;
> Till *Condon* for the Great Invasion fam'd
> Found out its use, and after him 'twas nam'd,

A less colourful but rather more likely explanation of the word is that it derives from the latin verb 'condere' (to contain), though in May 1985 yet another theory was advanced. The midwife responsible for the birth of the word was neither the Latin language nor the redoubtable (if legendary) Dr C. – a far more elevated being had his finger in this particular pie: God himself. According to this new etymology, condom is an abbreviation of the Latin phrase 'Cum Domine', with the Lord, that is, God! Presumably this was a prayer uttered by the users in view of the unreliability of contraceptive techniques, and may also date it to the period when condoms were used but not yet branded as blasphemous, possibly the sixteenth or seventeenth century. However, the wonderful new invention praised in the poems was not all that new – and possibly not all that wonderful. Madame de Sévigné, that indefatigable producer of the other sort of French letters, wrote to her daughter in 1671 that they were 'armour against enjoyment and a spider web against danger'. A century later her compatriot the Marquis de Sade wrote that he knew of three methods of contraception: the sponge, the sheath and anal intercourse. Naturally (or, what in his case was the same thing, unnaturally) the last method was the one he preferred.

Casanova, too, was an early user of what he called 'redingotes d'Angleterre' (English overcoats), 'that wonderful preventive against an accident which might lead to frightful repentance' (possibly VD), and 'the preservatives the English have invented to shelter the fair sex from all fear' (of pregnancy, obviously). In a Marseilles brothel he was offered a sheath which he found too coarse, and was then brought a selection of superior ones which were, however, only sold in dozens. Determined to get his money's worth, he asked for a fitting:

> The girl came back with the packet. I put myself in the right position, and ordered her to choose me one that fitted well. Sulkily, she began examining and measuring. 'This one doesn't fit well', I told her. 'Try another.' Another and another; and suddenly I splashed her well and truly.

Casanova seems to have been aware that the best method of testing a condom is to fill it with air, since one illustration from his biography shows him doing just this – though there is also a rather party-like atmosphere in the picture. What this does show is that in spite of his promiscuity, he did adopt a responsible attitude to his partners as well as a simple desire for self-protection, which seems to have been the main motivation in eighteenth-century England (warding off the 'Venus' Fire' mentioned in *Almonds for Parrots*).

This was certainly the case with Dr Johnson's crony and biographer, James Boswell. His *London Journal* for 1763 contains a

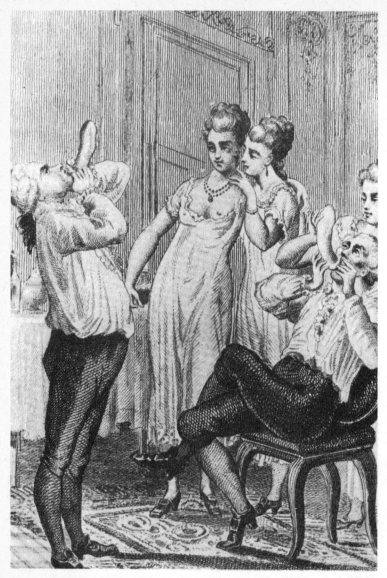

5. Casanova (1725–1798) testing condoms. Although he didn't like them – it was like shutting himself 'in a piece of dead skin' – he did use them as a contraceptive.

number of very frank entries concerning his sexual activities. Having already been infected by a woman whom he had assumed to be virtuous (before her 'seduction' by him), he determined to be more careful, and on the 25th of March we find him in St James's

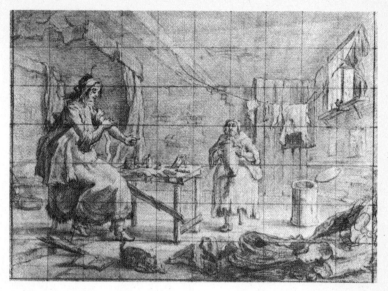

6. Hogarth's Harlot, with condoms lying on the table. Like other 'Industrious Jennies', she could quite likely have washed them after use and resold them to unsuspecting clients.

Park where he 'picked up a whore. For the first time did I engage in armour, which I found but a dull satisfaction.' In spite of this, discretion remained the better part of valour, and on the 31st he 'strolled into the Park and took the first whore I met, whom I without many words copulated with free from danger, being safely sheathed. She was ugly and lean and her breath smelt of spirits. When it was done, she slunk off. I had a low opinion of this gross practice and resolved to do it no more.' Like most such resolves, however, it didn't last long. By the 10th of May he was at it again on Westminster Bridge 'in armour complete . . . The whim of doing it there with the Thames rolling below us amused me much.' By the 17th he was over-confident again: 'I picked up a fresh, agreeable girl called Alice Gibbs. We went down a lane to a snug place, and I took out my armour, but she begged that I might not put it on, as the sport was much pleasanter without it, and as she was quite safe. I was so rash as to trust her, and had a very agreeable congress.' The next day, on the other hand, 'much concern was I in from the apprehension of being again reduced to misery, and in so silly a way too.' On June 4th he has returned to the use of precautions, this time wetting the condom (in a canal!), probably to enhance the fit. This method was certainly known to William Pattison, a Fellow of Sidney Sussex College, Cambridge:

MARY PERKINS, ſucceſſor to Mrs. Philips, at the Green Caniſter in Half-moon-ſtreet, oppoſite the New Exchange in the Strand, London, makes and ſells all ſorts of fine machines, otherwiſe called C———MS.

Dulcis odor lucri ex re quâlibet.
De quel coté le gain vient.
L'odeur en eſt toujours bonne.

Alſo perfumes, waſh-balls, ſoaps, waters, powders, oils, eſſences, ſnuffs, pomatums, cold cream, lip-ſalves, ſealing-wax.—N. B. Ladies' black ſticking-plaiſter.

NUMBER XVII.

WHEREAS ſome evil-minded perſon has given out hand-bills, that the machine warehouſe, the Green Caniſter, in Half-moon-ſtreet in the Strand, is removed, it is without foundation, and only to prejudice me, this being the old original ſhop, ſtill continued by the ſucceſſor of the late Mrs. Philips, where gentlemen's orders ſhall be punctually obſerved in the beſt manner, as uſual.

N. B. Now called Bedford-ſtreet; the Green Caniſter is at the ſeventh houſe on the left hand ſide of the way from the Strand.

7. A handbill from Mrs Perkins's condom warehouse, where she 'makes and sells all sorts of fine machines' and 'N.B. Ladies' black sticking plasters'!

Of Parent Wave, from whence it came,
Still mindful, the *Idalian* Dame [Aphrodite],
Ordains it shall all Sizes fit,
Provided that it first be wet;
And when put off to End of Time,
Should smell of *Fish* and feel of *Slime*.

Long before the advent of the London Rubber Company, in the middle of the eighteenth century London seems to have been the centre of a thriving international condom trade. The two doyennes of the business were Mrs Philips and Mrs Perkins, who as well as conducting their trade also conducted a propaganda war against one another in their handbills. Mrs Philips opened her warehouse at the sign of the Green Canister in Half Moon Street. Business went so well she sold out to Mrs Perkins, but within ten years was back again, selling from the sign of the Golden Fan and Rising Sun near Leicester Fields a great choice of skins and bladders, to 'apothecaries, chymists, druggists &c.', and supplying 'ambassadors, foreigners, gentlemen and captains of ships, &c. going abroad . . . with any quantity of the best goods in England, on the shortest notice and lowest price.' She also claimed to have received large orders from 'France, Spain, Portugal, Italy, and other foreign

Mrs. PHILIPS, who about ten years left off bufinefs, having been prevailed on by her friends to reaffume the fame again
upon reprefentations that, fince her declining, they cannot
procure any goods comparable to thofe fhe ufed to vend ;——
begs leave to acquaint her friends and cuftomers, that fhe has
taken a houfe, No. 5, *Orange-court*, near *Leicefter-fields*, one
end going into *Orange-ftreet*, the other into *Caftle-ftreet*, near
the *Upper Mews-gate*.——To prevent miftakes, over the door is
the fign of the *Golden Fan* and *Rifing Sun*, a lamp adjoining
to the fign, and fan mounts in the window, where fhe con-
tinues to carry on her bufinefs as ufual.——She defies any one
in *England* to equal her goods, and hath lately had feveral
large orders from *France, Spain, Portugal, Italy*, and other
foreign places. Captains of fhips, and gentlemen going
abroad, may be fupplied with any quantity of the beft
goods on the fhorteft notice.

8. A handbill from the 'real' Mrs Philips, 'maliciously reported . . . dead', railing
against a 'most infamous and obscene handbill or advertisement' put out by a 'mere
imposter'.

places', and had an advertising jingle, which in those enlightened
days she was not prevented from using (though, of course, they had
no TV either):

> To guard yourself from shame or fear,
> Votaries to Venus, hasten here;
> None in our wares e'er found a flaw
> Self-preservation's nature's law.

People in eighteenth-century England were certainly aware that the
condom could prevent conception as well as disease, as we see in
these lines from *The Machine* (1744):

> By this Machine secure, the willing Maid
> Can taste Love's Joys, nor is she more afraid
> Her swelling Belly should, or squalling Brat,
> Betray the luscious Pastime she has been at.

That this was not necessarily obvious can be seen from the following, written by a German doctor in 1906: 'This method is said to be
disadvantageous for the wife, since it makes it impossible for sperm
to enter the uterus'. Precisely!

The Opposition Musters

But Thomas Aquinas's words of warning had not been totally

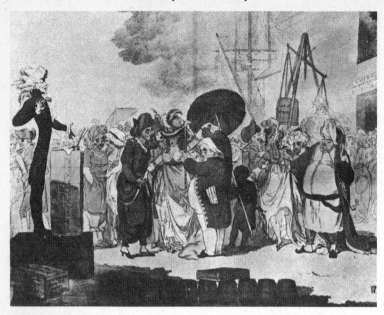

9. James Gillray's 'A Sale of English Beauties in the East Indies', 1786, shows just how far Mrs Philips's wares travelled: the auctioneer's block is a parcel of condoms from her warehouse.

forgotten in the Christian West. As long as condoms were only meant to prevent infection, they were permitted, and few found anything wrong with them. After all, the pillars of society could not be laid low by syphilis, could they? We already know that condoms were only available to the upper classes because of the expense – and they decorated them in all kinds of ways; though not with pictures, as William Pattison again tells us:

> The interceptive Shield they bear,
> Fit only too for love to wear:
> On this, no Images are plac'd
> (. . .)
> Lest the rough Surface damp the Sense.

A far cry from the decorative variety of modern French Letters, or even Victorian London. Hector France describes a visit to Petticoat Lane in the 1880s:

> Everything can be found there. Jewellery. . .watches, pornographic cards and French Letters with the portraits of Prime Minister Gladstone and Queen Victoria.

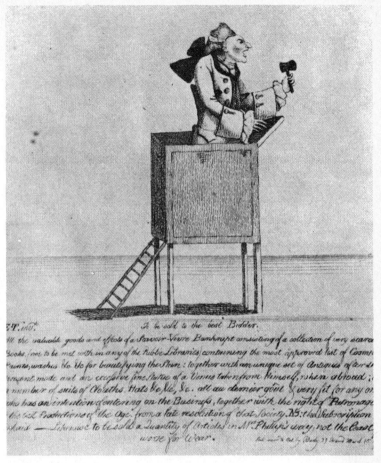

10. Another print by Gillray, 1773, 'To be Sold to the best Bidder . . All the valuable goods and effects of a Scavoir-Vivre Bankrupt', which seems to include 'a Quantity of Articles in Mrs Philips's way, not the least worse for Wear'.

Have we discovered a new (and very apt) idea for Royal Wedding souvenirs?

In 1952 a quantity of late eighteenth-century skin condoms were found in a locked box in an English country house. They were in three sizes, and double wrapped in packets of eight. Dr Dingwall of the British Museum examined them and reported:

> The specimen submitted is apparently made from some animal membrane and, as far as could be discovered, seamless, the edge of the open end being turned over and roughly stitched with cotton to form a hem

through which is threaded a strip of silk. Its approximate dimensions are: length 190mm, diameter 60mm, thickness 0.038mm.

This last compares more than favourably with the modern condom, whose thickness is approximately 0.07mm.

Still at the British Museum, and lovingly stored in a section known as the 'Secretum', are two fine examples discovered in the adjacent British Library in 1953 – also examined, it seems, by Dr Dingwall. Dated at between 1790 and 1810, they had for a number of years been pretending to be bookmarks. However, their origins must remain clothed in mystery to avoid unnecessary embarrassment to the owner's descendants – the books in which they were found came from the library of an Archbishop.

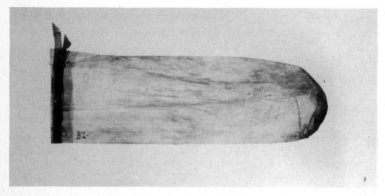

11. One of two sheep-gut condoms stored in the British Museum's 'Secretum'. The colour of vellum, and paper-like, this one still has the original red ribbon used to hold it in place.

Their manufacture was a complicated (and no doubt messy) process. Gray's *Pharmacopoeia* of 1828 describes how it was done:

> Condoms, Armour, Baudruches, Redingotes Anglaises [though by the 1847 edition this last had become French Letters]. The intestina caeca of sheep soaked for some hours in water, turned inside out, macerated again in weak alkaline ley changed every twelve hours, scraped carefully to abstract the mucous membrane, leaving the peritoneal and muscular coats; then exposed to the vapour of burning brimstone, and afterwards washed with soap and water: they are then blown up, dried, cut to the length of seven or eight inches, and bordered at the open end with a riband: used to prevent venereal infection, or pregnancy.
>
> *Baudruches fines.* The blind guts are soaked in weak ley, then turned inside out, and dressed as before: soaked again in ley, brimstoned, drawn smooth upon oiled moulds of a proper size, observing that the external coat of the gut is next to the mold, and dried.

There were also *baudruches superfines* which were 'scented with essences, and being stretched on a glass mould, rubbed with a glass to polish them', and *baudruches superfines doubles,* which were a sandwich of two of the superfine model. One can see why they were so expensive!

Still, even though only the upper classes had access to them, they were being called 'unChristian' and 'immoral' as early as the eighteenth century. While Boswell and his lady friend were dallying on Westminster Bridge, the forces of reaction were already mustering to spoil their fun. However, the pro and contra condom groups can't be divided along any clear social lines.

On the one hand there were the morally outraged who rejected contraceptives for Christian motives. After all, the Bible tells us to go forth and multiply, doesn't it? (It also tells us to replenish the earth, not overpopulate it, but that's another matter.) Another group can also be found in the same boat as the Bible fanatics, and they are the hypocrites, like Joseph Cam who wrote in 1734 that 'to publish methods of prevention smells so rank of the Libertine and Freethinker that it ought not to be allowed in a Christian country'. Or, reading between the lines, it's all right to do these things as long as you don't talk about it. Those who know about it can carry on – and who knows about it? Why, the upper classes, of course!

This view was a very tenacious one: Mary McCarthy's girls in the bestseller *The Group* discuss contraception in the 1930s and come to the conclusion that they should be available to the responsible middle classes, but not to the workers and other plebs.

The workers themselves did not share this view at the beginning – at least not the working women. In England and France (in Germany and Scandinavia everything happened later, and there's not such good evidence) handbills about birth control were being distributed by peddlers at the beginning of the nineteenth century. A Commission investigating the dissemination of 'obscene publications' reported that in 1834/5 600 copies of three books on contraception had been sold in Manchester, and no doubt the information contained in them was spread by word of mouth, thus reaching an even wider public. This seems to have been the case even earlier in Yorkshire, where an MP, on hearing from a textile worker that fewer illegitimate children were being born, asked: 'Do you mean that certain books, the disgrace of the age, have been put forth and circulated among the females in factories, to the effect you state?' 'Yes.' 'And you attribute the circumstance of there being fewer illegitimate children to that disgusting fact?' 'Yes.' How many books the peddlers actually distributed, we do not know – nor if they actually peddled contraceptives as well.

The Opposition Spreads and Flourishes

In 1798 an up and coming young economist by the the name of
Thomas Robert Malthus published a book entitled *An Essay on the
Principle of Population*. In this work he propounds the theory that
poverty and misery are a direct result of excessive population
growth. His basic idea is that the human race expands more quickly
than we can increase the production of food. According to Malthus,
the solution to this problem was to be found in wars or plagues, and
in preventive measures such as late marriage, sexual abstinence and
contraception (though this last was considered by him to be a
'vice'). The work was a considerable success and the grateful establishment appointed him Professor at the East India Company's
Haileybury College. His theories were still the subject of controversy right down to our own century. Seen from a late twentieth-
century perspective which includes Ethiopia for example, he wasn't
totally wrong – but he wrote more than just warnings against over-
population. He believed that the natural order of things meant that
a lot of people should be poor, and a few should be rich, as there was
by no means enough to go round. However, if the population
continued to grow, the poor would take more and more for themselves while still remaining poor, and the rich would simply become
poorer. This was obviously a shocking and unacceptable idea, and
so he demanded that the poor should stop breeding like rabbits.

Among the middle classes his ideas fell on fertile ground, and
even some workers were convinced by them. Francis Place, a self-
taught tailor and radical who knew about the appalling conditions of
working-class life because he had been born in a debtors' prison,
wrote his 'Diabolical Handbills' under Malthus's influence. Place
was also one of the first people to try, with superficial medical
justification, to regulate human sexual behaviour. He laid down
once and for all who could do what and with what and to whom (and
even when they could do it!). Transgressors would run the risk of
appalling physical and mental punishment. For example, women
who remained 'abstinent' (presumably by abstinent he meant in-
tact) until the age of 26 were threatened among other things with
diseases of the uterus. In London he handed the handbills out – in
the company of John Stuart Mill, who is not unknown to feminists –
in market-places and to people on the streets, and they were also
distributed in the North of England. However, no mention is made
in them of our friend the condom, possibly because its cost would
have been too great for the workers the leaflets were aimed at. One
of the Place's followers, Richard Carlile wrote *Every Woman's
Book, or What is Love?* in 1825, and he actually says 'The sponge is
the female's safeguard; but there are other means, by which con-

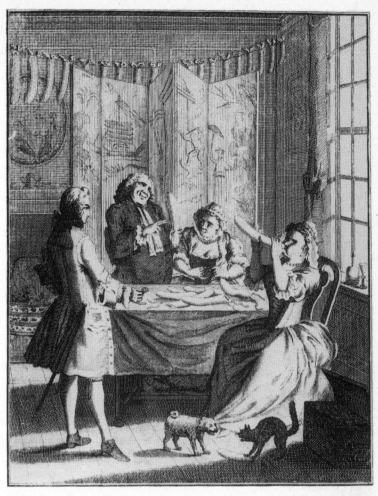

12. The frontispiece from the 1744 edition of *The Machine; or, Love's Preservative* showing a condom warehouse. Note the range of sizes available to customers. Once again the condoms are being tested in the age-old manner.

ceptions are avoided, to be practised by the male. One is to wear the skin, or what in France is called the *baudruche*, in England commonly the *glove*. These are sold in London at brothels, by waiters at taverns, and by some women and girls in the neighbourhood of places of resort, such as Westminster Hall(!).' But he is not very much in favour of the condom, which he seems to regard as 'artificial or unnatural' as compared with the sponge. His book, incidentally, caused a certain amount of scandal because it was pub-

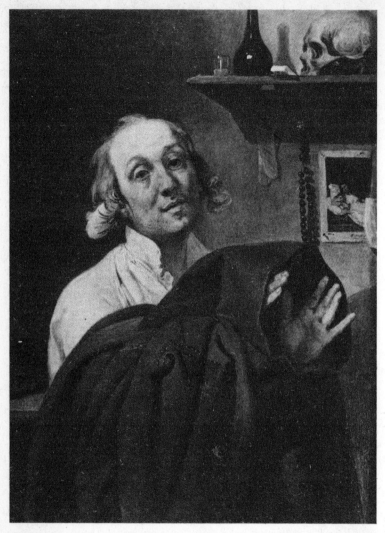

13. A self-portrait by the German artist Zoffany, 1779. His condoms are hanging the right way up under the mantlepiece.

lished at the same time as a cookery book of the same title, which must have confused would-be cooks and birth controllers equally. Both Place and Carlile were prosecuted, not to say persecuted, but we must admit that the reasons were as much to do with their radical political beliefs as their advocacy of contraception.

This all shows how schizophrenic the debate about contraception had become at that time: the workers should be persuaded to stop breeding, that was officially acceptable; but attempts to help them to do this were frustrated if not punished.

Most of the workers' leaders were fanatically anti-Malthusian, though. His teaching seemed to them – with every justification – to be an attempt by the ruling classes to shirk their responsibilities, to prevent reforms and to consolidate their hegemony. On the other hand, anti-Malthusian voices could be heard among the middle classes as well. If the workers were no longer forced to devote all their efforts to saving themselves and their ever-increasing families from starvation, they might start using their surplus energy for riot and revolution. And this seemed worse to many of them than Malthus's nightmare visions, which didn't directly affect them in any way. For their part, the workers refused to allow anyone to stick their noses (or anything else) into their reproductive habits. The catchphrase 'The right to choose' was relevant even in those days – except that it was men and not women who were demanding it.

So we find a number of strange bedfellows at the beginning of the nineteenth century. On the one hand, a number of middle-class population experts, some workers' leaders, a few radicals and the early feminists: obviously in favour, if not always of French Letters, at least of contraception. On the other, the Christians, the hypocrites, the majority of the (male) workers' movement and a few members of the middle class who were concerned about their property: equally obviously against. A somewhat confusing state of affairs.

Virtue Triumphs

While this debate was still raging, the development and exploitation of the colonies was progressing by leaps and bounds. The rubber trade in South America expanded, and in 1844 Mr Hancock and Mr Goodyear, now immortalised in tyre advertisements, invented the vulcanisation process. From now on it was possible to manufacture rubber condoms, which had two big advantages: they could be stretched, and they were cheaper than sheep-gut condoms. But they were still expensive, especially for those who needed them most, so it took a number of years before the French Letter became a genuine item of everyday wear.

The early rubber sheaths had a seam, rather like that on a stocking, whose contribution to the pleasure principle was negative rather than positive. They were of two basic types: first, the common or garden condom that we all know and love. It has no special name and is regarded today as the 'normal' condom. A doctor, himself a member of the nobility, described it early in the twentieth century in the following poetic manner:

> The condom consists of a delicate membraneous tube which corresponds to the dimensions of the erect penis, is sealed at the front end and at the rear end usually has a fastening device (ribbons).

How unimaginative modern condoms seem in comparison! They are sealed, admittedly, but there is no fastening device at all. We can never go to a fancy-dress party wearing a condom instead of a false nose – a choice which was available to our grandmothers.

In England, rubber condoms were traditionally made in three sizes, and its US cousin, in only one.

The second basic type was the tip condom, which, as its name suggests, covered only the glans. Its inventor describes it as follows:

> When filled with water, the condom has the shape, either of an egg from which a small section has been cut, or of the glans penis. At the open end the membrane is thicker and forms a ring which holds it on. When the condom is in use this ring fits so tightly around the glans that the condom cannot slip off during intercourse, since the ring cannot pass the corona glandis.

He then concludes that 'the tip condom is preferable to all other known contraceptives'. Well, he would, wouldn't he?

Nowadays they are known as American tips and are more a curiosity than anything. In the early days they were unpopular because they didn't provide enough protection against infection, and couldn't be produced and bought as anonymously as other kinds of condom. A tip condom had to be tailor-made so that it could neither slip off nor constrict the penis. So before buying a tip the penis had to be measured by the doctor to find the right size, and then you had to ask for the exact size when buying them: just the same procedure a woman has to go through to obtain a diaphragm – but who ever heard of a man who was willing to undergo so much hassle? Perish the thought.

The rubber condom had hardly started on its triumphal progress, however, before the doctors who wrote about it developed a sensibility unknown to their colleagues in earlier centuries:

> Just imagine having to remove the condom after every passionate embrace. What bliss, what poetry is trampled underfoot! And yet the aura of poetry, of the mysterious is of the greatest importance, especially in the marriage bed, less for the sake of the embraces themselves than for everyday life together.

Still, in spite of seams, tips and sensibility, no less a figure than George Bernard Shaw hailed the rubber condom as 'the greatest invention of the nineteenth century'.

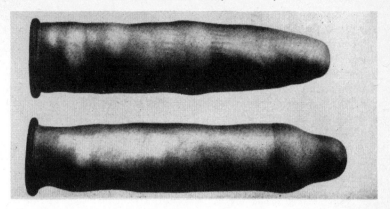

14. Two rubber sheaths, included to show just how far condom technology has progressed since those uncomfortable days (and nights).

The Condom and its Adversaries: Peaceful Co-existence

Even the invention of the rubber condom and its increasing popularity didn't cool the ardour of its adversaries. The Malthusians began to publish their own books (one of which, published in 1887 had the bashful title *The Wife's Handbook* and, moreover, gave the wrong timing for the 'safe' period); and the feminists, who didn't want to be lumped in with the Malthusians, agitated for women's right to self-determination. For their part, 'honest and upright' citizens feared the total decay of morals if contraceptives were available to all. What was sauce for the gander was still not sauce for the goose: when Annie Besant in 1877 published an American work on birth control called the *Fruits of Philosophy* (a rather mild work, recommending the douche as the best method), she and Charles Bradlaugh, her co-publisher, were prosecuted in London for:

> . . . unlawfully and wickedly devising and contriving and intending . . . to vitiate and corrupt the morals as well of youth as of divers other subjects of our said Lady the Queen, and to incite and encourage the said subjects to indecent, obscene, unnatural and immoral practices, and bring them to a state of debauchery, therefore . . . did print, publish, sell and utter . . . a certain indecent, lewd, filthy, bawdy and obscene book, called 'Fruits of Philosophy' . . .

The jury found that the book was obscene (it did, after all, contain a diagram of the female genitalia) but exonerated the defendants from any corrupt motive in publishing it. This didn't prevent them from being found guilty, but the conviction was overturned on a technicality after an appeal. All of which did Annie Besant no good:

she was later deprived of her child because she was considered
morally unfit to care for her.

The doctors also wished to get in on the act, and began to
fulminate against contraceptives on the grounds that they were
unhealthy – which most of them except the condom certainly are.
But these doctors claimed to have found side-effects totally different from the ones we know today. C H F Routh in 1878, calling birth
control 'sexual fraudulency and conjugal onanism [masturbation]',
said that it induced in females:

> death or severe illness from acute and chronic metritis, leucorrhoea,
> menorrhagia and haematocele, histeralgia and hyperaesthesia of the
> generative organs, cancer . . . ovarian dropsy and ovaritus. In cases
> where severe results are not observed, the organs become so over-
> changed that sterility results from their chronic disease. Lastly, mania
> leading to suicide and the most repulsive nymphomania are induced.

Men, too, were at risk – of mania, loss of memory and suicidal
urges. However, the fact that the good doctor's fears may have been
moral rather than medical emerges later on, when he asks of
husbands:

> If you teach them vicious habits, and a way to sin, without detection,
> how can you assure yourself of their fidelity when assailed by a fascinat-
> ing seducer, and why may not even the unmarried taste of forbidden
> pleasures also: so that your future wife shall have been defiled ere you
> knew her?

Nevertheless these prophesies of doom could not really harm the
French Letter. Not even Marx and Engels managed that; because of
course these two gentlemen also wished to join in the debate. They
naturally saw the whole thing from an anti-Malthusian viewpoint
(they used to call him 'that detestable Malthus'). Engels was prepared to admit that even a communist society might one day see
itself forced to take contraceptive measures to prevent over-
population, but that would be decided by the people themselves.
For this reason he was opposed to the enlightened writings of his
feminist female comrades. He apparently advocated – if he could be
said to have advocated anything at all – abstinence rather than
contraception, if only to avoid having to agree with the detestable
Malthus's League on a single point.

And the Lawyers?

They mostly confined themselves to confiscating informative
books about contraception and dragging their authors before the
courts. The hypocrites were at work even here: laws against contraceptives were reserved for the twentieth century. The nineteenth

century merely wished to ensure that they weren't mentioned in public. In this way the spread of information about contraception was hindered, but those who knew about them could always get hold of them.

The USA was the one exception to the rule as a result of the activities of Anthony Comstock, Secretary of the Society for the Suppression of Vice. In 1873, contraceptives were forbidden, as was the dissemination of information about methods of contraception through the post. The noble condom was, however, excluded from this ban, being labelled as a preventor of infection: it then became a medicine and were made subject to the regulations of the Federal Drugs and Food Administration. For almost a hundred years condoms could only be sold in the USA with a warning on the packet that they were 'For disease prevention only', an association that still lingers today and one that has traditionally given the condom a bad name.

As the nineteenth century drew to a close, the adherents of Marx and Malthus continued to hate each other's guts; but the condom was firmly set on its throne, and humanity was grateful for its existence.

The Twentieth Century

One of the greatest early revolutions of the twentieth century – less famous, but no less important, than the Russian Revolution – has most unfairly never been celebrated in song, story or on the silver screen. Several poets have been asked to write a revolutionary canto or two in its praise, but not a line has turned up as we go to press. This revolution took place in the realm of the condom – as in so many others, the time was ripe at the turn of the century: it became possible to make seamless and therefore more comfortable condoms. In order to achieve this long-desired effect, glass moulds were dipped in a liquid rubber solution. The same method made the production of condoms with a teat at the end. In a word, the tried and trusted friend we all know so well is as old as the century. The next revolution occurred in the thirties, when the latex method was invented. The instigators of both these revolutions remain anonymous. Latex is the proper name for the sap of the rubber-trees. Previously, this had to be made into rubber and then into condoms. Now condoms could be produced directly from latex, and as a result became simpler and cheaper to manufacture.

The advantages of the latex method must surely have convinced the last remaining doubting Thomases: the condoms that resulted lasted much longer than the old ones. Then it was only three

months, but today it's said to be two to five years. The experts are
not all in agreement about this: no one has offered to leave their
French Letters unopened for that long.

Perhaps the mystery could be solved by the Irishman who fell
red-handed (and red-faced) into the hands of the Irish Customs
towards the end of the seventies with a lorry-load of 40,000 condoms: this led to a very complicated court case: basically, all contraceptives were forbidden, but they could be provided on prescription
or imported for personal use. A doctor only had to write such a
prescription if his conscience would allow him to. The chemist in the
same way only had to fill the prescription if his Christian and
Catholic conscience would permit. In small towns especially, it was
impossible to get one's hands on a sheath at all. So when the said
gentleman was caught with his 40,000 condoms he swore to high
heaven that they were all intended for his personal and private use.
Now even the Irish gardai have other things to do than worry about
the destination of 40,000 condoms, and so they let him go. But then
the press started to do their sums: with a shelf-life of five years at
most, how many condoms a day do you have to use to get through
40,000 condoms before they (or you) perish? There were also the
female journalists who, just before condoms were legalised, were
trying to make a programme about the absurdity of the Irish laws.
When they turned up at the border the customs man just waved
them through. This was not at all what they wanted, and after
several protests, they managed to persuade him that what they were
doing was illegal, so they drove back into Northern Ireland and
returned, cameras running. 'Now', said the bold exciseman, showing his best profile, 'I'm afraid you can't bring those into the
Republic.' But they were all luckier than one protestant Kerry
doctor. Customs in Cork impounded four dozen condoms which he
had ordered by post from England. They sent him a letter saying
that such articles in this quantity must be imported personally,
accompanied by a satisfactory verbal explanation concerning their
intended use (Christmas decorations, perhaps?) to safeguard
against illegal sale. While the dispute was going on, the doctor's
wife became pregnant.

Your man's acquisition of 40,000 French Letters was made possible by another advantage of the latex method: the production of
condoms had now been automated. The conveyor belt has thou-
sands of glass moulds 35cm long and 35mm in diameter. These are
first dipped into liquid latex, pass through a dryer, and back into
liquid latex: a process that is repeated until a film 0.07mm thick has
been built up. The open end is rolled up by brushes, thus producing
the ring at the end, then off into hot air chambers for vulcanisation.
Finally the condoms are powdered and carefully unrolled from the

moulds. With automation production was increased and prices lowered. They were more elastic than before, and needed less storage space, which provided a big advantage when transporting large quantities.

We have now arrived at the type of condom which is the norm today. Everyone thinks it's so ordinary and natural that older types (fish-bladder, sheep-gut) are often looked on as a joke, even by the most experienced French literateurs. Of course things are always developing. Condoms are getting thinner, are being lubricated with spermicide, flavoured, made in horned and rippled shapes (though no longer, alas, with the pretty ribbons of yesteryear). And at another level of development progress is also being made: in safety.

Condoms and Safety

Around 1930 complaints were still being made that 50–60% of condoms were faulty. It is obviously difficult to be absolutely certain about such statistics: had anyone ever seen a man turning up in a chemist's shop or a factory with a burst condom in his hand and asking for his money back? Imagine taking the French Letter back immediately after the accident. You might prefer to wash it first, but then the manufacturer would claim the damage had happened while it was being washed. Certainly not while it was being used. 'A condom from our factory? Never. Easier for a camel to pass through the eye of a needle!'

Anyway how are you going to prove it was the condom that was faulty and not your technique? And what are you going to produce as evidence? After all, no condom manufacturer guarantees their products are 100% failsafe. As far as we know, there has never been a successful case conducted against a condom manufacturer for failure of goods, and this is probably why liability insurance for people in the condom business is low. Even if you can produce irrefutable evidence of condom failure, like the two healthy twins an American couple did, you're still not home and dry. They filed a suit against both Schmid Laboratories who made the offending article and the chemist who sold it to them. Schmid, quick to assert their rights, immediately sued the couple for negligent use of the condom. (Unfortunately they had not had the foresight to film the episode, paying close attention to thrashing genitalia, as they weren't that sort of couple.)

Things really went wrong when they contested that Schmid could contersue them, as this involved attending a court in New Jersey, where their apppeal was overruled. This not only gave the local papers a field day, but the local radio and TV network as well. It didn't do a lot for the couple concerned, especially when the media revealed that they were members of a religion that prohibited the use of contraception anyway. Fearing the consequences of the publicity and possible disciplinary action from the church (who must have got a lot of pulpit mileage out of God's mysterious ways), the couple abandoned the suit, settled for a small sum and were left not holding one but two babies, and a media reputation they're still trying to live down. Somehow we don't think they will ever use a 'Fourex' condom again as long as they live.

Undoubtedly, today's condoms are safer than their predecessors – but our forebears left no stone unturned when trying to ruin the reliability of their condoms. The high percentage of condom failures in the thirties didn't come about because people were less reluctant to wave their torn condoms about in public. Nor is there any truth in the rumour that the Government (or the wicked capitalists) employed someone in each factory to make holes in every tenth French Letter to keep the population up and the workers down. In those days there were no electronic tests either. If faulty condoms didn't come to light in the factory or in the field (a sociologist's way of saying 'in use'), the researcher had to invent other methods. So the poor French Letter was subjected to all kinds of stresses and tortures by this scientific inquisiton – and the lay user was recommended to do the same.

A popular method was to blow them up, just like a balloon – a pastime that is still popular today. Then the inflated condom was held up against illuminated frosted glass, felt carefully by hand and closely watched. It was thought even better to fill it with tobacco smoke and press the smoke into all parts of the condom. A condom can also be filled with water; but with all these procedures you run the risk of doing too much of a good thing and bursting – or even worse, weakening – your condom.

Using these methods it's hardly surprising that 50% of condoms failed the test in 1930. In fact, it seems to speak for, rather than against, the quality of French Letters in those days. Modern researchers are of the opinion that these methods probably brought about the demise of more condoms than the most careless manufacturing methods could produce.

Another reason for the frequent failure of these early condoms lay in faulty use. One doctor, for example, felt it necessary to give his readers the following warning as they climbed between the conjugal sheets: 'Accidents can also happen if you do not put the condom on before penetration takes place'. It wants no ghost, come from the grave, to tell us that!

And the Opposition – were they Silent?

No, not at all, but – apart from extreme cases like Ireland – it didn't do them much good. And the Irish example shows us the special position of condoms: they are the only contraceptive which is easy to use, not dangerous to your health, and easy to transport and conceal – at least in quantities less than 40,000 (if this seems a lot, by the way, you should remember that the average factory produces up to 72 million condoms per annum and LRC Products Ltd, manufacturers of '██████', 150 million condoms). You can add to this the useful fact that the condom also protects against infection, a service no other contraceptive can offer.

The opposition seems to have accepted this by the turn of the century, at least most of their supporters did; but the hypocrites continued their activities in both word and deed. While few outside the churches and of course the medical profession actually opposed the existence of condoms, open discussion of them (or any other contraceptive method, for that matter) was forbidden or suppressed. This meant that when birth control clinics and advice centres were opened, many had to use rather ambiguous names, like the 'Walworth Women's Welfare Centre' opened in 1921. This did, however, help to protect the women using them (then as now the patients were mainly women) from public scandal – that this was likely can be seen from the experience of workers at one such centre who had to run the gauntlet of jeers and shouts of 'whore!' on their way in to work. One such centre which opened near Manchester had the advantage of being situated behind a pie shop. No one could be sure if the women were buying the family lunch, or making sure that they had a small enough family to afford one at all.

The first clinic and advice centre was opened by Margaret Sanger in Brownsville, New York in 1916. She was a radical socialist who had started a magazine called *The Woman Rebel* in 1914. This trumpeted forth ideas like 'the marriage bed is the most degenerating influence on the social order' and listed the rights claimed by the Rebel Women: the right to be lazy, to be an unmarried mother, to destroy, to create, to love, and to live. Their duty was 'to look the whole world in the face with a go-to-hell look in the eyes; to have an ideal; to speak and act in defiance of convention'. The magazine announced that the law on contraception would be defied, and Margaret Sanger published a pamphlet called *Family Limitation*. Both its strident political views and its advocacy of contraception made the magazine intolerable to people like Comstock, Secretary of the Society for the Suppression of Vice, and because of this and the pamphlet Mrs Sanger was held to have violated nine federal statutes. She escaped to England the day before the trial.

Here she met Havelock Ellis who encouraged her to concentrate on birth control rather than waste her energies on so many disparate causes. She also met Marie Stopes (of whom more soon), though what actually transpired in the relationship between these two strong-willed women is obscured by their later disagreements, particularly on Margaret Sanger's side. While she was avoiding prosecution, the radical Emma Goldman, who had been lecturing on birth control in America for years, began to discuss the subject more openly than before: she was arrested, fined and imprisoned for distributing birth control literature. Margaret Sanger's husband was also arrested and brought to trial late in 1915 for distributing her pamphlet. But changes had been taking place in the US: in March 1915, a group of Liberal women had founded the National Birth Control League, and among other things were demanding a change in the law:

> The League specifically declares that to classify purely scientific information regarding human contraception as obscene, as our present laws do, is itself an act affording a most disgraceful example of intolerable indecency.

Margaret Sanger returned to America and was not prosecuted for her previous offences. She continued to defy the law, founding the New York clinic in 1916. Long queues of women collected, and within ten days the Vice Squad (of all people) arrived and arrested the staff. One of them, Ethel Byrne, went on hunger strike and was pardoned and released after 11 days, because she seemed so near to death. Margaret Sanger was released on bail, and immediately re-opened the clinic. The police were just as quick to re-arrest her, charging her with 'maintaining a public nuisance!'; she served thirty days in prison for this awful offence. But it was only a matter of time before birth control advice became legal, although the last of the Comstock Laws was repealed as late as 1966.

In Britain, there were no laws specifically prohibiting contraception or contraceptive literature, though the latter was often prosecuted under the laws applying to 'obscene' publications. Contraceptive knowledge was spreading, too. This can be seen from a comparison of the birthrates of two London boroughs; Shoreditch (a poor East End area) and Hampstead (predominantly middle-class) had roughly the same rate of births per 1000 in 1881 (31.2 and 30.0 respectively). By 1911, the Hampstead birthrate had fallen to 17.5, but in Shoreditch it remained at 30.2, again an indication of the class-bound nature of contraceptive information. The First World War also made a difference: it was possibly the issue of condoms to the army that made them familiar to members of all classes, becoming the most popular method of birth control. A survey done in 1946/7 showed that of the 15% of those married before 1910 who used some form of birth control, and the 40% of those married 1910–1919 who did so, by far the majority used the sheath. However, the spread of knowledge was hit-and-miss, and depended a lot on advertisements, some of which were for products that were not effective or reliable. Clearly there was a need for something in England similar to Margaret Sanger's clinic.

Enter, to fill this great gap, Marie Stopes. Although she remained a life-long opponent of the device this book is celebrating, declaring it to be 'harmful' (though it is not clear to whom), her contribution to the history of the birth control movement in Britain cannot be ignored. Her first marriage was not very successful: it took her own research in the British Museum to discover that after some time of marriage she was still *virgo intacta*, so she had the marriage annulled in 1916 on the grounds of non-consummation. Still a virgin, she published in 1918 *Married Love*, a book intended to help others avoid her mistakes and have a happy and enjoyable sex life. The astounding information that women might actually enjoy sex (in spite of the denials of both the Victorians and certain modern groups) could have been one cause of its success – it sold 2,000 copies in a fortnight). It contained only the briefest reference to contraception so, in response to letters begging her to remedy this lack, she published *Wise Parenthood* later in 1918. Even those in the medical establishment who were in favour of some forms of birth control were not prepared to accept works published so openly – and by a *woman* who was not even a medical doctor. One of them described her books, mild though they would seem compared with today's marriage manuals, as 'practical handbooks of prostitution'. Undaunted by this criticism, and heartened by the support of so many whom her works had helped, Marie Stopes, with moral and financial support of her second husband Humphrey Roe, opened the first British birth control clinic at 61 Marlborough Road, Holloway, on 17 March 1921. The Mothers' Clinic for Constructive Birth Control was intended to reach out to those women, particularly of the lower classes, who were ignorant of the difference birth control could make to their lives by freeing them from the burden of unwanted pregnancies. She made it clear that she was not against children as such (in fact, she was very much opposed to the economic arguments of the Malthusians). What she wanted was freedom, sexual satisfaction and the chance for joyful motherhood for all women: an ideal that still seems utopian 66 years later! Among the positive elements of her clinic was the waiving of charges to those who couldn't pay, helping to reach precisely those who needed the information most.

C.B.C.
THE MOTHERS' CLINICS
OF THE
Society and Clinic for Constructive Birth Control and Racial Progress

President :
MARIE CARMICHAEL STOPES, D.Sc., Ph.D., F.L.S., F.G.S.

Vice-Presidents :

COL. R. J. BLACKHAM, C.B., D.S.O., M.D.
ROBERT BLATCHFORD, ESQ.
THE VISCOUNT BUCKMASTER
THE REV. H. G. CORNER, D.D.
THE RT. HON. THE EARL OF CROMER, G.C.B., P.C., etc.
MRS. PERCY DEARMER
SHAW DESMOND, ESQ.
LADY DUCKHAM
LADY CAREY EVANS
MAJOR SIR THOMAS CAREY EVANS, M.C., F.R.C.S.
PROFESSOR HENRY PRATT FAIRCHILD, U.S.A.
SIR RICHARD A. GREGORY, D.Sc., F.R.S.,
          LL.D., F.R.Met. Soc., F.Inst.P.
ARTHUR L. HUMPHREYS, ESQ.
SIR FREDERICK KEEBLE, C.B.E., M.A., Sc.D., F.R.S.

COUNCILLOR E. KING, J.P. (Ex-Mayor of Islington)
SIR W. ARBUTHNOT LANE, BART., C.B., M.B.
MRS. PETHICK LAWRENCE
THE REV. H. D. A. MAJOR, D.D.
PROFESSOR BRONISLAW MALINOWSKI
THE RIGHT HON. LORD MARLEY, D.S.C., J.P.
SIR GEORGE MITCHESON, M.P.
ALDERMAN J. S. PRITCHETT, M.A., B.C.L.,
                          Recorder of Lincoln
MISS MAUDE ROYDEN, C.H., D.D.
DR. G. R. ROSS
LT.-COL. SIR WILLIAM A. WAYLAND, J.P.,
                          F.C.S., F.S.A., M.P.
PROFESSOR E. A. WESTERMARCK, PH.D.
MRS. ISRAEL ZANGWILL

Hon. Secretary :
HUMPHREY V. ROE, ESQ.

Hon. Treasurer :
A. S. E. ACKERMANN, ESQ., B.Sc.(Eng.), F.C.G.I.

Hon. Solicitors : MESSRS. BRABY & WALLER, Dacre House, Arundel Street, Strand.

Bankers : MESSRS. BARCLAYS LTD., 262, Tottenham Court Road, W.1.

106, WHITFIELD STREET, TOTTENHAM COURT ROAD, LONDON, W.1

SPACING BABIES FOR HEALTH
The Use of Condoms
(Popularly called Sheaths or French Letters).

The fundamental teaching of our President and the Mothers' Clinics has been that contraceptives used by the male are less physiologically right than the best type used by women. The C.B.C. Committee is still strongly of the opinion that where possible the wife should be properly fitted at a Clinic with the contraceptive best for her own use.

Some people are so placed that they cannot visit a Clinic immediately after marriage. Moreover there is no clinically recommended feminine method which can be used by virgin girls, and so brides cannot be reliably fitted until a few weeks of marriage have passed. These, and other factors in our social life sometimes make the use of the condom by the man temporarily advisable.

The commercial trade in condoms is generally profiteering, and often has unpleasant associations. For many years the C.B.C. Society, disliking their use, left patients coming to its Clinics unhelped regarding condoms.

As exposed in the House of Commons Debate recent commercial developments have become so offensive that the C.B.C. Committee, after mature consideration, decided that it would be failing in its duty if it did not make it possible for those needing help to obtain through its irreproachable source reliable and inexpensive condoms.

Every type has been tested most carefully and the C.B.C. now supplies really satisfactory thin condoms or sheaths.

Packets of three for 1/-
(Postage 2½d.)

The C.B.C. Committee considers that these condoms at three for 1/- will solve many of the problems which have unfortunately accumulated round the provision of this type of contraceptive.

Special price to Doctors £1. 18. 0. for a gross Condoms (in packets of 3).

Cash with order.

15. A 'Constructive Birth Control' leaflet, reluctantly advising the use of condoms (Marie Stopes was personally opposed to them). More interesting is its attack on the condom suppliers: clearly there wasn't an Office of Fair Trading then!

During the twenties, apart from continued opposition, particularly from the Roman Catholic church and some diehard doctors, the situation gradually improved. Oppositon within the Church of England had effectively been silenced by a speech made by Lord Dawson, George V's personal physician, to the lay Church Congress in Birmingham in October 1921: instead of supporting the backward-looking bishops, he startled them by supporting contraception and saying 'Birth control is here to stay. It is an established fact, and for good or evil has to be accepted . . . no denunciations will abolish it.'

The Catholic press and some Anglican bishops attacked him, the *Sunday Express* thundered 'LORD DAWSON MUST GO', but by and large comment was favourable, and this unequivocal support from an establishment figure was later claimed to be 'one of the most important events in the twentieth century history of birth control'.

The year 1930 was a watershed for both good and ill. First, the bad news: Pope Pius XI issued his encyclical *Casti Connubii*, on the duties of Christian marriage. Artificial contraception was shameful, intrinsically immoral and an unspeakable crime. (At the time he was probably referring to withdrawal and the condom, though his successor Pius XII extended it to include diaphragms and douches, leaving only the 'safe' period – Vatican roulette, as it has come to be known.) And this, particularly under the conservative régime of St Peter's current successor, is where the Church remains today, at least officially, causing the misery of 'sin' and guilt to those who do use contraceptives, and untold miseries to many of those who don't – as well as their proliferating offspring.

The good news in Britain was the foundation of the National Birth Control Council (later the Family Planning Association). The pressure which led up to this had also prompted the Minister of Health to issue Memo 153/MCW which, while still erring very far on the side of caution, made it possible for local authorities to establish what were, in effect, birth control clinics. Our friend Johnny shared in the good news in 1932 when a survey showed that the sheath (plus a spermicide) was the most reliable method of contraception followed, in order of reliability, by the Dutch cap, the cervical cap and withdrawal.

Not everything was so rosy abroad: faced with a vast population loss during the First World War France outlawed contraception in 1920 (the years after were known as 'les années creuses' – the hollow years – during which whole areas were practically depopulated of young men, or indeed any men at all). In Germany, contraceptive advertising was forbidden in 1922 (without much success), and the Nazis forbade all contraception in 1933. After all, the country needed soldiers and mothers of soldiers – those who were unworthy of that dubious honour were sterilised and didn't need contraceptives. But as we observed earlier, the soldiers who were needed also had to be protected against streptococci, and so we find 'Arian' businessmen taking over rubber companies previously owned by Jews. Of course, they prodcued other things as well, but they didn't stop making condoms: one of them even had a letterhead showing a condom box and boasting that the firm was no longer in Jewish possession.

Opposition to the condom also came from the moral front. In Norway, the evils of the 'New Morality' were inveighed against: 'The New Morality does not seek to conceal that what it wants is to enable people to sin and be merry'. And who wants merry sinners? We don't have the phrase 'as miserable as sin' for nothing, do we? Birth control, like everything new, was seen to be the last straw which would break the floodgates and bring the end of family life, morality and civilisation as we know it. No one stopped to consider whether a civilisation which could be destroyed by as little a thing as a condom was worth having.

The supporters of the condom now ceased to try and tempt potential users by promising enhanced pleasure, but instead took to stronger measures, such as knocking copy against our old friend Coitus Interruptus (withdrawal, to his English friends):

> If the penis is withdrawn before ejaculation, the duration of peripheral stimuli is shortened, and perhaps because of the use of the will-power to interrupt coitus, the nerves which hinder erection come into action at the wrong time. The nerve material of the group of muscles which cause ejaculation is harmed, as is their effectiveness. During normal coitus the content of the seminal vesicles is expressed during the whole time of ejaculation into the pars membranacea (the rear part of the urethra), but in this case this process is disturbed, and the seminal vesicles, and perhaps even the vasa deferentia are not sufficiently emptied.

As if this were not horrific enough, the side-effects are even worse: nervous irritation, first of the spinal column, then the whole body, and finally, inevitable impotence!

Even if you haven't understood a word of this, it's obvious that withdrawal must be shunned like the plague, if for no other reason that women should be concerned with their lovers' health. [A sigh from the typist shows that she wishes that men would show the same concern for their lovers' health, and stop insinuating that the Pill and the IUD are so handy.] And carrying on without condoms not only has a bad effect on men's nerves – it's also hard on the women who have to bear the consequences. As another wise tome of that period points out, 'women have to make the greatest sacrifices during pregnancy' and:

While men are beginning to pay more heed to the sufferings and worries of women in this connexion, we must sadly admit that there are still too many reckless men who put their own selfish pleasure first. Drunkenness is still a problem in married life. And drunkennes and selfishness are an evil combination. Of course, if a man is paralytically drunk, he's not interested in coitus: and even if he were, he may not be capable. The danger is greatest when a man is just drunk enough to overcome his inhibitions: then he is willing to risk it.

Is he willing to pull a condom over it even when he's sober? But perhaps we should go along with those who regret that men are normally excluded from contraception, and believe in their basic good will (Is that a [male-chauvinist] pig I see flying round the room?).

Johnny Comes Marching Home

The Second World War brought a whole series of problems in its wake – several clinics in major cities were destroyed by bombing, for example – but one of the greatest was quite simply a shortage of rubber. The London Rubber Company at one stage actually made caps out of rubber sheeting which had been ordered for the bathroom floors of a Paris hotel – perhaps the first time decorated caps have been made. By 1942 there was an acute shortage of rubber, and people began to fear that supplies might literally be stretched too thin, resulting in sub-standard contraceptives. Roman Catholics called on the Prime Minister to stop the manufacture and suppress the sale of contraceptives 'in the interest of national welfare', but once again the need to protect the soldiery from disease prevailed, and supplies were made available to clinics. Since the war, the problem had been more one of education than anything else, though perhaps one should note the years 1964 (when the first Brook Centre for the *un*married was set up – the FPA had previously confined its advice to those who were married or about to be) and 1974, when the Labour Government finally introduced free contraception. Some sections of the popular press had a field day: LOVE ON THE NHS: 'CHAOS' (the *Sun*), but generally, in spite of administrative hiccups, the system began to work quite well.

Less so in Germany, perhaps, where in 1959 the sale of condoms in vending machines was prohibited. A minister called Würmeling (appropriately meaning 'little worm') was largely responsible. The regulations stated that 'Devices for contraception or the prevention of sexually transmitted disease may not be offered for sale in vending machines in public places, roads or streets'. Fortunately, an exact interpretation of the words of the text saved the slot machines:

to offer for sale (feilbieten) means to *display* for sale, and a toilet is not public in that sense. So vending machines were banished to dark lavatory corners (men's lavatories, of course, since the sale and purchase of condoms is men's business, according to a lot of people: and that is still the case, since there are still books which show condoms and the female genitalia – but without a clitoris!). In 1970, however, the highest Federal Court came to the decision that 'these devices are among those things which today can be regarded as acceptable and normal and in no way dangerous'; and in spite of opposition from Catholic Bavaria, that's the way things went.

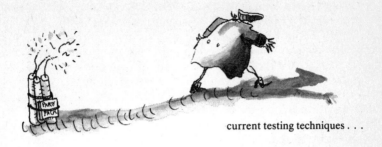

current testing techniques . . .

The Contemporary Condom

To get a clear picture of the current condom situation in the UK you need to transport yourself to the leafy suburb of Chingford where, secreted amongst the neat semi-detacheds, a giant condom production line spews out condoms in every shape and form around the clock. Within the confines of a discreet baby-blue building some 800 employees work wonders with latex, producing not just condoms, but rubber gloves (the 'Marigold' type), surgical and industrial gloves and contraceptive diaphragms. Could the popular expression 'no glove no love' as they quip in the States, have its roots in this mixed production line process one wonders.

The London Rubber Company

London International's Chingford plant ejaculates 100,000 condoms every couple of hours, up to 150,000 million a year of which 70% are exported. That still leaves a healthy 850,000 gross per annum to be consumed in the UK. Which means, on average, four times a second somebody's up to no good with one. A venture that started as a small importing business in a room in the city in 1916 has mushroomed into a multi-million pound organisation, whose brand name '█████' is so established in the British vocabulary, that it's become a generic term. Indeed, we understand that the next entry for condom in the *Oxford English Dictionary* will include it as such. '█████' is to condoms what 'Hoover' is to carpets. The London Rubber Company first started production in the thirties, but it was the Second World War, when it became the sole suppliers of condoms to the armed forces, that their prospect of becoming a household name was assured. Needless to say the condoms supplied

41

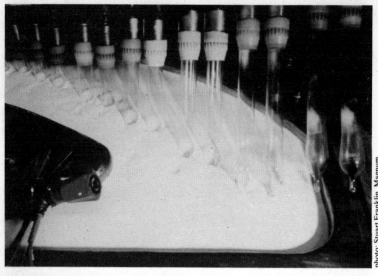

photo: Stuart Franklin, Magnum

16. Glass formers, the shape of condoms, being dipped in a swirling latex solution at London International's Chingford plant.

during the war were primarily to prevent the debilitating effects of VD rather than unwanted children. Thus LRC's reputation for a safe and reliable product was established and fears of august Catholics infiltrating production lines with pins were allayed. Not that this stopped vending machine graffiti. In the seventies, when the claim on condom machines was 'approved to British Standards' a common addendum was 'so was the Titanic'.

According to the Family Planning Association, condoms are 85–98% effective with careful use. LRC are not only stringent with their own testing, but are also subject to at least six visits a year by the British Standards Institute who conduct their own tests on production-line condoms. It is the approval of the BSI that provides each packet of LRC condoms with the kitemark that spells security and safety to the majority of condom users. At London Rubber the humble condom has to be subjected to a lot more than electric shock treatment to prove its worth. 'Electronically Tested' as LRC's products boast means easing a latex sheath onto a metal phallus, immersing it into a saline solution and passing an electric current through it; any imperfections will interfere with the sheath's insulation properties. Trained women, whose lives consist of metal phalluses and shock treating condoms, know exactly what to watch out for. In fact, detecting defective stock must be the highlight of an otherwise monotonous day. Once packed the condoms are kept under lock and key (just in case), which does make you wonder

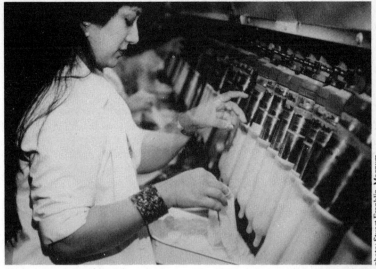

17. Electrically testing condoms in Chingford by slipping them onto metal mandrels, putting them into an electrolyte solution and giving them an electric shock.

whether perhaps there is an element of truth about sabotage on the condom front.

However, samples are subjected to even more gruelling tests than this, feats beyond the capabilities of the most athletic or well-endowed couple. For example, the average condom will stretch from eight inches to five feet (well beyond the realms of reality), will accommodate 40 litres of air (that's the equivalent of two buckets of water and they don't as far as we know, have much demand from elephants) and a one inch strip of condom latex will support over nine pounds in weight before breaking (presumably for obese sperm). On top of all this you will also find testers blowing them up to bursting point or rolling waterfilled condoms over blotting paper to find tell-tale leak marks.

London International Group's pre-tax profits on total sales for 1985/6 stood at £24.1 million, of which condoms account for 20% of sales. These profits are expected to rise to £28 million during 1986/7, and £33.5 million in the following year – no wonder they felt able to put in a £150 million takeover bid for Wedgwood china several years ago. When the manufacture of condoms is such a lucrative business, you may well wonder why there aren't baby-blue condom factories springing up all over the country.

The problem is that a monopoly situation prevails. LRC Products account for between 95% and 97% of total condom sales in the UK. Add to this the huge quantities exported and you begin to see the picture. LRC/LI make vast fat profits, so much so that they have twice been the subject of the Government's Monopolies and Mergers Commission investigations. The last Report in 1982 (Cmnd 8689) found their profits so large that it concluded 'the United Kingdom prices for sheaths may be expected to become excessive' and referred their prices for monitoring by the Office of Fair Trading. LRC's evidence at the time: 'There were no foreseeable developments that could bring a significant and sustained increase in demand so risk was all "downside"'! Clearly this no longer applies now that it has been confirmed that condoms provide protection against AIDS. As Kleinwort Grieveson Securities Ltd (*Investment Research*, January 1987) indicate, there will indeed be a marked growth of condom sales – perhaps by as much as 10% per year over the next 10 years – almost guaranteed by the Government's widescale 'safe sex' advertising campaign. (LI's shares have increased in value from 90p in 1985 to 259p in early 1987 and 407p in February 1987.)

This situation has already led Clement Freud MP to ask the Secretary of State for Trade and Industry whether he is satisfied with existing competition in the condom market, and if he has had many requests to refer it to the Monopolies and Mergers Commission.

Contenders in the Condom Market

In the UK, contenders like Michael Conitzer and his 'Jiffi' brand and Patrick Moylett's Prophyltex 'Red Stripe' condoms are very much fringe organisations. We the public are still insecure and suspicious about anything not named '██████' and not bearing a BSI kitemark – such is the effect of over fifty years of conditioning. But that is no guarantee a '██████' will be infallible. A friend of ours once had part of a sturdy LRC product removed at the doctor's surgery. surgery.

Competitors in the condom market come and go. Remember the 'Horizon' brand of condoms launched in the late seventies against '██████' – they finally threw in the glove in 1983. The latest contender for a slice of the market is 'Lifestyles', the brand that aimed to include women in the act with their 'Menswear for women' campaign. 'Lifestyles' are an American brand, distributed by Warner Lambert, the largest suppliers of over-the-counter chemist requisites in the country. You'd think they'd be able to make some dent in LRC's almighty latex coating, but in the two years they've been competing, they've been forced to lower prices and have currently stopped all advertising (could this mean they'll be with-

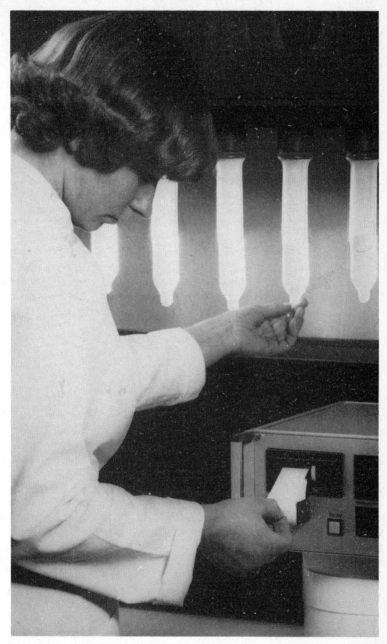

18. Testing for water leaks at a factory in West Germany. The BSI in the UK require that one per cent of all production is sampled and tested.

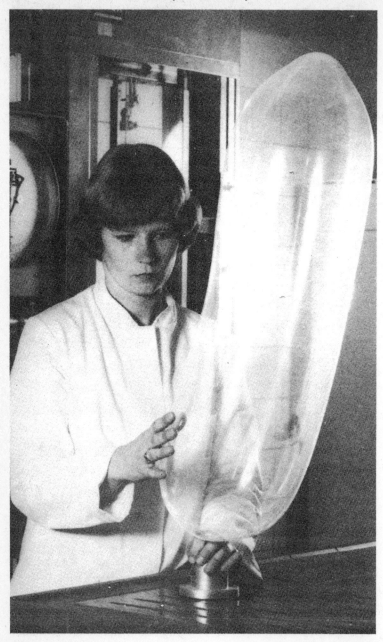

19. Inflating a condom to destruction in West Germany, a sure sign of any variations in wall thickness.

to launch a discreet new 3-pack this year, which means they are still willing to do battle on LRC's terms.

Meanwhile the two ultra-fringe contenders stick to their guns, and for the time being content themselves with a few humble slivers of the gigantic LRC cake. Both by sheer coincidence come from rag-trade roots. Michael Conitzer and the lively advertising slogans that accompany his products – like 'Real men do it in a Jiffi' – is in fact managing director of the Stirling Cooper retail womenswear chain of shops. Patrick Moylett was working in the fashion industry in Paris when, looking for a moneymaking scheme, he had the foresight to obtain licences from the leading German and French condom manufacturers. His first target however was Southern Ireland: when the buying of condoms on prescription finally became legal in 1980 Moylett was poised and ready to swoop. He bought 50 gross of French condoms, docked at Ross Lair and sold the lot in the first town he got to. Earlier entrepreneurs had not been quite so lucky.

Moylett gained a reputation in the tabloid press for being the 'King of Condoms' in Ireland, although he still had terrible problems advertising his mail order service, even in 1985 when they finally became available off prescription. His first advertisement was: 'Send £5 and receive two dozen condoms by return'. This was rejected on the grounds that the word condom was not permissible. Moylett then tackled the considerable problem of advertising a product without mentioning it. He finally settled for: 'Send £5 and receive two dozen French samples by return'. Now the normal enquiring mind might well think in terms of underwear or *pâté de foie gras* come to that, but the Irish Advertising Standards Authority decided that anything French must be naughty and anything naughty, of course, must be related to sex. Humph! He finally resorted to: 'Send £5 for two dozen samples'. This you'll be pleased to know didn't affect Moylett's sales, but it does from time to time cause a little confusion, and has been known to result in urine samples for pregnancy testing being sent to him through the post!

Moylett's main strength in the UK condom market is the introduction of the French Prophyltex brand, 'Red Stripe'. These condoms are considered stronger, don't have a teat style reservoir at the end, and unlike the majority of condoms have been promoted in the gay market and the prevention of AIDS (Acquired Immune Deficiency Syndrome). As London Rubber, ever cautious about its public image, have no inclination to veer from the staid and conservative audience they aim their advertising towards, Moylett has jumped into the gap in the market. The 'Red Stripe' condoms, better suited to anal intercourse by virtue of their strength alone, are recommended (like all extra-strong condoms) by the Terrence

Higgins Trust, and are available by mail order, through vending machines at gay venues and through many of London's special clinics. Ridiculous as it may seem, they are not yet available on the NHS. Moylett is also attempting to make inroads into the general UK market with other Prophyltex brands, but is once again faced with the might of a monopoly, and the competitive prices LRC are able to tempt retailers with.

Michael Conitzer imports his 'Jiffi' condoms from West Germany, where they are categorised as medicines and undergo equally as stringent testing as they do in the UK. Conitzer argues that LRC condoms are overpriced. As he points out: 'I can bring them in from Germany for 2p each, the pack costs me 7p plus 3p for printed material. So a pack costs me 30p and I sell them for £2, I've quadrupled my profit margins.' We will add that Conitzer is laughing all the way to the bank, but not at the intended expense of the public. He first tried selling his condoms for £1 for ten but no one wanted to buy them. Unfortunately price and quality are synonymous, doubling the price doubled his sales.

Conitzer, approaches the sales and marketing of condoms in exactly the opposite way to LRC. His condoms come in designer packs: sleek black flip-top cigarette-style packets, dispensed from refurbished Wurlitzers and old-fashioned cigarette vending machines, anywhere he can put them. Youth clubs, pubs, gay venues, and in his Stirling Cooper boutiques. He's even positioned one outside his King's Road branch for easy access. His main audience is the teenage market from 13 years upward (LRC don't target anyone under 16, in spite of the fact that 33,000 abortions were carried out on girls under 19 in England and Wales in 1984).

Conitzer reckons condoms have to be enticing and attractive. He gives teenagers exactly what they want, and makes purchases as painless and accessible as possible. 'Jiffi' brands include party colours, Benzocaine-tipped varieties that numb the penis and delay premature ejaculation, and ribbed condoms for extra sensitivity. Conitzer also targets the gay market, advertising regularly in the gay press (an area the '████' brand neglects), and arranging distribution at gay venues. His up-front marketing includes 'Jiffi' sweat-shirts and T-shirts with full instructions on how to use a condom on the back. Both Conitzer's and Moylett's approach to condom marketing are guaranteed to cause apoplexy amongst the moral majority, but then unwanted pregnancy and the stemming of sexually transmitted diseases, especially the AIDS virus, must take priority. Maybe the market leaders will learn from their approach.

Advertising and Packaging

As any advertising executive working on a condom account will tell
you, finding a way to spread the word about your product can be a
tricky business. Advertising is currently banned on both TV and
radio, and press advertising is at the discretion of the editor of the
publication. Sex, you see, is a taboo subject and one that embar-
rasses us so much that we cannot bear to be reminded of it during
our average night's TV viewing – even though a commercial might
appear between some explicitly sexual film like 'Body Heat', or
indeed a programme about contraception. These peculiar double
standards are of our own making and are confirmed in a survey
conducted by the IBA (Independent Broadcasting Authority), who
govern advertising on radio and TV, in October 1980. 61% of
people interviewed said they would indeed be offended by contraceptive advertising. (Surprisingly, even countries like Catholic Italy
have a more liberal attitude than this.) So, given the narrow scope
available, when Tony Hodges and Partners Ltd took over the
'Lifestyles' account, they did indeed find themselves with a problem
on their hands. Press advertising was immediately discounted. Fleet
Street tabloid editors may well use scantily clad provocative female
pin-ups to sell their papers, but they don't want to embarrass their
readers with condom advertising. Therefore most condom advertisements, outside of soft porn magazines, are discreetly honed
down to calling-card details. As a consequence, advertising is
bland, circumspect and mostly devoid of the sexually illicit humour
which might appeal to a younger audience or encourage a change in
practise.

   The agency opted for a national poster campaign. The 'Lifestyles'
advertisements were benign and totally inoffensive, depicting a
young couple with caption lines aimed specifically at women:
'Menswear for women' and 'Lifestyles, the male contraceptive
women will prefer'. South London feminists did substitute castra-
tion for 'Lifestyles' at one particular site, but in the main the
campaign was inoffensive to the majority of the population, with
the exception of British Rail and London Transport who bluntly
refused to take them. They did, however, take the provocatively
sexual 'Pretty Polly' tights' advertisements that offended women
from one end of the Northern Line to the other.

   London Rubber Company also know the problems of attempting
an innovative approach to sales. Their controversial racing car
sponsorship in the seventies so offended the sensibilities of the BBC
they refused to cover the race. Yet without the help of the most
powerful media it's almost impossible to reach high-risk groups like
teenagers and the gay community. AIDS shows no sign of a let-up

and at the present time no cure. The only permissible advertising on TV and radio is for general contraception, with referral to bodies like the FPA or to a GP. The sort of people we should be preaching to, however, are not the converted and not those likely to want to tell their GP or the FPA about their sex lives. As the censors' veil is lifted on another taboo subject – menstruation – the situation becomes even more ironic. We can now watch without embarrassment advertisements for sanitary towels and tampons, but not the one item that will ensure a regular flow.

The current government TV advertising campaign to create public awareness of AIDS and its prevention does now make a reference to condoms, keeping in step with its posters and leaflets. However, it is already clear that the £20 million allocated to the overall campaign this year will not overnight make up for the many years of self-censorship practised by the media. AIDS has come face to face with the contradictions of our Victorian past, and the question is whether a cure will be found before we have to recognise our human sexuality openly and honestly – not as something smutty and unspoken. Journeyman's survey found that 72% of all male participants thought there should be advertising on TV and radio, and 71% of the women. 79% of the men agreed that condoms should be more easily accessible to the under-16s, and 93% of the women. Clearly the majority are in favour of both advertising and making it easier for under-16s to get condoms (the women, of course, are more enlightened!). But both sexes are more cautious about advertising, reflecting just those contradictions inherent in British morality. As Philip Meredith at the IPPF (International Planned Parenthood Federation) says: 'Britain could be far more adventurous in promoting contraception, particularly amongst the young' and cites the seventies Swedish sheath campaign as an example of more progressive attitudes. Aimed specifically at the youth market, it was witty (with condoms depicted as funny faces) and poignant. Their campaign included TV commercials, and the results showed a drop in unwanted pregnancies, a levelling-off of abortions and a decline in gonorrhoea. Between 1970 and 1980 when the Swedes were effectively halving their VD rates, here in the UK we were actively propagating it and doubling our figures.

But even Swedish tactics can't beat Thailand's approach where Mechai Viravaidya has earned himself a Peace Medal from the United Nations for his amazing feats performed on the contraceptive front. Mechai effectively reduced the population growth in a ten year period from 3.3% to 1.9%, and has also made substantial inroads into the problem of VD. Mechai, being an economist, saw exactly how too large a population and the debilitating effects of sexually transmitted diseases can interfere with the economy. He

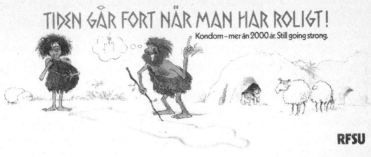

20. Upfront condom promotion in Sweden. The main headings, freely translated, read: 'Time flies when you're having fun'; 'Watch out for lovebugs'; the bottom one should be self-explanatory.

certainly didn't waste his time pandering to the Victorian attitudes of the conservatives. He designed and executed probably the most up-front condom assault the world has ever seen. He blew up condoms on TV and organised condom blowing-up competitions for children and conducted a 'Cops and Rubbers' campaign, issuing the whole of the Bangkok police force with rubber protection. Mechai's message was so powerful and effective he even got religion on his side, with local Buddhist priests sprinkling consignments of condoms with holy water to demonstrate their approval. So successful was the campaign that 'Mechai' now means 'condom' in Thailand. Whether President Reagan appreciated Mechai's inauguration greeting 'Blessings of the subdued fertility' (along with a card for a free vasectomy in Bangkok) is not known. The offer, although kindly, was probably offered a little late in the day for the ageing septuagenarian.

But for sheer ingenuity and volume, it is the Japanese (the largest consumers of condoms in the world), who merit a special mention. As far back as 1977, some 79% of all fertile Japanese couples were using condoms as their main form of contraception. We might add here that this impressive statistic is not entirely due to the allure of latex, but partly due to the illegality of the contraceptive pill (other than on medical grounds for menstrual disorders), and partly Japanese culture. The Japanese do not take kindly to chemicals or foreign bodies floating around their systems, interfering with their ying and yang. Even so, taking all this into account, it's still a hefty total. It is also interesting to note that they have a very low percentage of AIDS victims – only 26 reported so far, of whom 18 have died, out of a population of 121 million.

Another relevant factor must surely be the way in which condoms are promoted and sold in Japan. To begin with distribution is widespread, supermarkets everywhere carry stocks, conveniently placed next to womens' sanitary goods, as it is Japanese women who are the main condom buyers. Vending machines are also common, although there were initial problems with children mistaking them for bubble-gum machines (which probably put a lot of Japanese children off bubble-gum for life). In Japan, distribution is so widespread that women even sell condoms door-to-door – one brand was actually packaged to look like an encyclopaedia. Advertising and packaging promote not only the efficiency of the goods but the added pleasure and erotic potential of the condom. Brand names reflect this, with titles like 'Lady Wet'!

The Japanese, rather like the French, find the UK package-of-3 mentality risible: they sell condoms in realistic quantities of 25, 50 and even 100. Furthermore packaging is as attractive and tempting as possible. Leading Japanese commercial artists are employed to promote condoms in the same way as any other household items, and novelty packaging, accessories and gimmicks are all part of the incentive to buy. You can buy condom packs disguised as cigarette boxes or as packs of cosmetics, some condoms even have musical

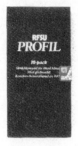
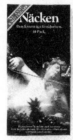
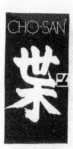
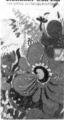
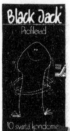
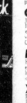
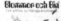

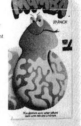

21. Swedish poster advertising different brands. The main heading is quite explicit: 'Sow in our seed-bags' and the packaging is bright and cheerful as well.

movements activated when the packet is opened. (Whether tunes are humorous like, 'If I'd known you were coming I'd have baked a cake', or serious like, 'I just can't help falling in love with you', we

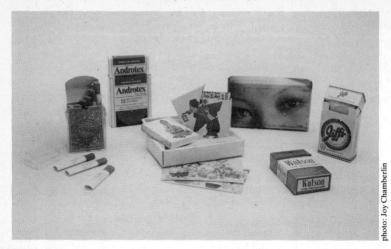

photo: Joy Chamberlin

22. Examples of unusual Japanese packaging. Each 'cigarette' on the left contains a condom; one of the woman's eyes winks when looked at from one side, and as the individual packets inside the box are opened an innocuous scene changes to one with sexual undertones. Is this meant to get you in the right mood?

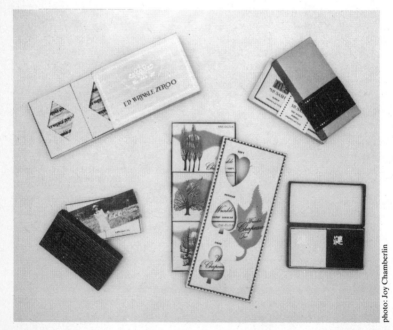

photo: Joy Chamberlin

23. The standard form of Japanese packaging. Nearly all are disguised to look like boxes of bath salts, are colourful, and often given names which are highly descriptive.

don't know, but we'd certainly like to get our hands on a pack.)

However, it's not just the packaging that's original but the contents as well, with every colour, texture and shaped condom you can imagine and the whole gambit of special features – like one brand of specially-contoured condoms that have little dotted lines up the front to ensure you put it on the right way, or condoms complete with tear-off boot style tags at either side so you can pull your condom on in style. Added accessories include thoughtful little disposal bags, and supplies of freshettes to clean up the equipment afterwards. As for colours, the Japanese have a preference for pastels like 'opal' to invite sweet dreams, 'pink' to promote a delectable mood, or exotic black. There are even psychedelic condoms to attract the youth market.

And what do we get here? Plain dull skin tones, and packages which at best promote 'Mills & Boon' style romance ('Lifestyles'), and at worst panoramic seascapes of sailing boats at sunset ('████') that have no obvious connections with sex at all. Some incentive!

The Feminist and the French Letter

Whatever the packaging, from a woman's point of view the condom is a fantastic contraceptive. It leaves responsibility for contraception to the man. It also protects us from a growing number of possible malaises, mostly on the increase because of alternative methods of birth control. In this field the Pill is the main culprit, and the side-effects of using it have in themselves done an admirable 'public relations' job for the humble condom. If you use the Pill there is no barrier between your vagina and cervix and the man's penis. Good thing too I can hear the hedonists shouting. Not all men wash themselves everyday, so *we* can understand only too well the lyric of Norwegian songwriter Kari Svendsen: 'Should I ever get married, it must be to a man who can be kept easily clean'. In an ideal world we wouldn't want anything to come between you and your pleasure, but by removing the barriers you're inviting all sorts of potential problems. Both cancer of the cervix and breast cancer have been linked with the Pill, there is evidence that cardio vascular disorders are associated with it, and its boom years correspond with an increase in sexually transmitted diseases.

And what are you increasing your chances of nurturing? Well, there is syphilis, gonorrhoea and all those VD-related infections, and of course there are warts and Herpes, which has of course now been upstaged by AIDS (Herpes might be painful, unpleasant and incurable but it is not going to kill you). There is firm evidence to support that using a condom will help protect you from all these ills,

including the latter. It has few side-effects, apart from the rare
rubber allergy (LRC has recently launched a special condom which
should help sufferers of this allergy), and it won't make you put on
pounds or feel like throwing up all the time.

Gay Condoms and AIDS

A homosexual, as the word implies, is mainly concerned with his
sexuality which he pursues with like-minded men in an homogenous
zone.

Unlike the heterosexual population, gay men do not don condoms to prevent pregnancy, but to prevent the spread of sexually
transmitted diseases. As far as we know, although condoms were
not invented by a gay guy, they were using them as far back as
Biblical times. Note Psalm 18, line 35 in the *Old Testament* where
David says: 'Thou hast given me the shield of Thy salvation and Thy
right hand hath holden me up, and Thy gentleness hath made me
great'. No question about what was going on here, or that the
'Shield of Salvation' was a condom from the Lord for David.

Historically, gays have been very quiet about their use of condoms, in the same way they have been quiet about their sexual
preferences, for fear of persecution, and indeed prosecution by
rigid societies. So we don't know a great deal about condom usage
and the gay market historically. A Doctor Magnus Hirschfield did
attempt in the thirties to research condom usage amongst gay
Berliners, but was obviously so carried away with the subject he
omitted to notice the rise of fascism. This was a gross, and unfortunate, oversight on his part, as it resulted in his expulsion from Berlin
and a public burning of all his valuable research material. Furthermore Hirschfield died in 1935, so we'll never know what it was he
uncovered.

One thing we do know about gay men and condoms, is that their
usage has increased considerably in the past few years. In 1979 there
was just one case of AIDS reported in the UK. By 1984 the number
had crept up to 36 and by early 1987 a disquietening 686 victims had
been registered. Meanwhile in the USA, where the virus was first
identified, current statistics stand at over 30,000 recorded cases with
at least one million people infected. In New York alone it is estimated
that one in two gays have been infected, a third of whom are likely
to develop the disease. Often derogatorily referred to as the 'Gay
Plague', the gay community are once again being unjustly persecuted
for spreading a disease that moralists see as 'divine retribution' for
the 'wages of sin'. In the words of James Anderton, Chief Constable
of Greater Manchester, people at risk from AIDS are 'swirling

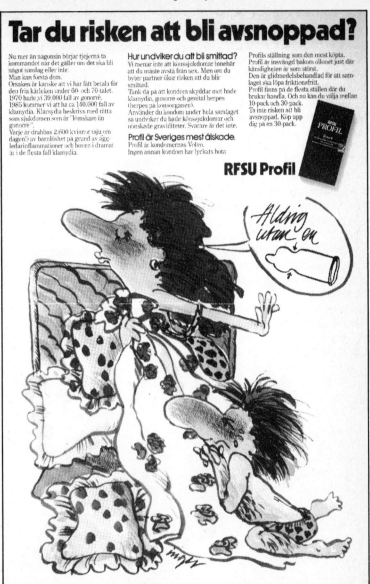

24. Another Swedish poster: 'Are you going to risk being rejected?' Her response to his pleading is 'Never without a condom'.

around in a human cesspit of their own making.' So before we continue we'll set the record straight. To quote Dr Robert Gallo of the National Cancer Unit, Bethesda, Maryland, USA: 'AIDS was never a homosexual virus. It's just that the homosexual group were the first to be infected in the USA'. Words of wisdom. In some African countries where homosexuality is uncommon, the AIDS virus is so widespread doctors are unable to single out any one high-risk group.

Meanwhile, all over the world the AIDS panic is on. In Bahrain for example we've heard all men and women have to pass an AIDS-free blood test to prove their purity. And apparently customs officials have been known to corner any likely-looking gay men and ask them confidentially if they've ever known Rock Hudson. In their confusion over the subject they appear to assume that AIDS came directly from Rock Hudson and not via Africa. In Los Angeles lawyers are busy drawing up legal contracts. If you want to bonk there these days you'll have to sign a document accepting financial responsibility for any nasty little germs you might pass on to the contract wielding man or woman concerned. Sex, it would appear, is getting a lot less spontaneous for both sexes, and can only continue to do so as the AIDS virus spreads to the heterosexual community.

AIDS is transmitted by an exchange of bodily fluids, and that, in the main, means from sexual intercourse. You can't pick it up from sitting on loo seats, sharing cups and glasses, or simply from standing next to a victim. But if you are an active gay guy (and we don't

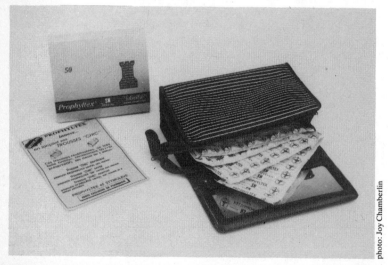

25. The sophisticated approach! A toilet bag containing 50 Prophyltex 'Red Stripe' condoms. Attractive to look at, and functional as well, but what do you do with a collection of toilet bags?

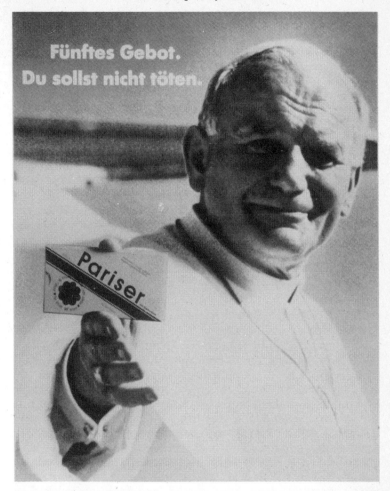

Fünftes Gebot.
Du sollst nicht töten.

Pariser

26. Photomontage of the Pope promoting condoms – used by the Swiss *Sonntags-Blick* newspaper during a campaign against AIDS and referring to the Fifth Commandment 'Thou shalt not Kill'.

mean not passive), or a heterosexual, come to that, it's only sensible to take precautions. Using a condom will help protect you against the whole gambit of nasty sexually transmitted diseases – including the terminal varieties. In the panic that hit San Francisco when AIDS first became known, condoms sold out, gays were advised to abstain from sex altogether, bars and saunas closed and weren't allowed to open up again until they started to distribute condoms free of charge. In the USA the rubber industry supports the AIDS help-groups.

In the UK the picture is very different. As late as April 1986 LRC were still denying that a condom afforded any protection against AIDS, and they certainly weren't advertising their products in the gay press. At the time of going to press LRC's policy regarding the gay market remains the same, with no prospect of them launching a specifically gay sheath, although they are currently testing a 'Duo' sheath in Holland. Clive Kitchener, director of LRC Products, when asked about the issue in *Marketing* (January 1987) commented: 'I don't think anybody likes to be labelled X, Y or Z . . . We would like to treat people as human beings'. Perhaps someone should point out that human beings are currently being treated for AIDS. Instead, it's been left to their fringe competitors to promote the condom to the gay market. Both 'Jiffi' contraceptives and 'Red Stripe' distribute to gay bars, clubs, bookshops and venues and advertise their services in the relevent media. 'Red Stripe' are also available at many of London's Special Clinics.

Current Standards

As far as the top ten condom manufacturers in the world go, the UK rates fourth largest, only bettered by China, Japan and the USA (this doesn't take into account that Japan and the USA include at least three manufacturers each, and the UK only one – which actually owns one of the American companies). It makes sense for condom manufacturers to ensure their products are tested accurately, as with all businesses the main motivation is profit. In this country we tend to be grossly insecure about buying any other brand but '███'. And yet there are many alternatives that are just as efficient, and some of which are cheaper. Just because a condom doesn't have a British kitemark, doesn't mean it's of inferior quality. Many brands will have already passed stringent tests in their country of origin, like the USA, and the manufacturers are just unwilling to pay extra for a British Standard, when their own standard is just as good.

Fortunately this problem over standards will soon be solved when the ISO (International Standards Organisation) eventually agrees (well, they've been thrashing the problem out since 1974) about acceptable standards across the board. The main bone of contention latterly has been agreeing on how to test a condom's strength, whether it's better to stretch a small piece of latex until it breaks, or whether it's more effective to inflate the manufactured condom until it bursts, or better to fill them with water. These are the questions they are asking themselves! Whatever the outcome you can be sure that when this International Standard comes into operation the products, and there will be an awful lot more of them, will all have been tested to the hilt not only for durability and lack of holes, but for colourfastness, secure packaging *et al*. They will also be a uniform length, thickness and width.

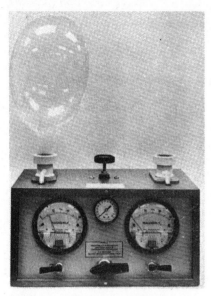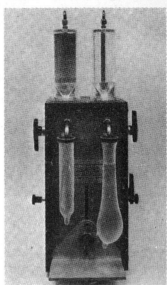

27. Two machines used by the PIACT in the USA to test condoms. The left tests for pressure and volume at bursting point, and the right for water leaks. The standard test is to fill the condom with 300ml of water, let it hang, close the end and roll it over chemically-sensitised paper.

But be warned, though, condoms only last for two to five years under optimum conditions. In an experiment conducted by PIACT (Programme for Introduction and Adaptation of Contraceptive Technology) in July 1980, it was discovered that condoms deteriorated when exposed to ultraviolet light. After as little as four to six hours exposure they burst more easily (perish the thought), and two of the unfortunate testers experienced failure rates as high as 50–75%. So heat and light can certainly limit the pocket or wallet life of your condom, not to mention the consequences of keeping your rubbers in the glove compartment of your car in a heatwave. All the more reason to buy your supplies in those neat dense aluminium wrappers and not in the transparent packs that some imported condoms come in. Following this train of thought you may well begin to wonder about condoms produced by Third World manufacturers, and what may be happening inside crates of condoms sweating under a midday sun as they wait to be sent on their way. Food for thought indeed!

Those of you who doubt the perishability of latex, can always conduct your own experiment. Take one condom, place in a sunny spot and leave for one month (for the sake of propriety we recommend using a new rather than used item, especially if placed in a well-frequented spot). Return in one month and your sample will have metamorphosed, out of all recognition, into a crisp brown Autumn leaf.

Another good way to lessen a condom's life, and a far more common one probably, given our lousy weather, is to use 'Vaseline' or any other petroleum-based substance as a lubricant. Although this may enhance the movement, it also weakens the latex. Stick to 'KY Jelly'.

So, if you use a bit of common sense, or should we say condom sense, there's no reason why you shouldn't already be playing the condom field in total safety. It's far more likely it'll be you rather than the condom that makes the slip-up at the end of the day.

International Condoms

Throughout the world, condoms are gaining in popularity. According to estimates by the Johns Hopkins University in late 1982, there were 40 million users worldwide, a quarter of whom were Japanese (in the UK no more than 1.3 million currently use our little friend, compared to nearly 3 million women on the Pill). From earlier figures, less than 1% of total users were in Africa, only 3% in Latin America, and 13% in Asia outside of Japan and China.

It is hardly surprising, then, that Japan produces a third of the 5000 million condoms manufactured each year which, if you have an agile mind, means that the Japanese user averages sex three times per week. Clearly this can't be true . . . and of course it isn't! They only buy 864 million condoms for their own use, which means a much more realistic twice a week – the rest are exported to countries like India. And to confuse matters further, India already produces enough condoms for its own needs, and exports to the Soviet Union and Eastern Europe. So to cope with this 'imbalance' India is doubling its production to 710 million condoms per year, and plans to double that again by 1987/8.

In Africa, where AIDS has long been established but often officially denied, the condom will come into its own, in a manner of speaking. The Kenyan Government now provides free condoms on demand, but the central issue for developing countries remains a question of mass education and cost. Without increasing subsidies throughout the production-distribution-retail chain few rural Africans are able to afford enough condoms to make any sense of local and international efforts to prevent AIDS from spreading across the entire continent. This, of course, draws us into the politics of condomology, and the effect huge donations of condoms by organisations like the United States Agency for International Development can have on the manufacture and marketing of condoms in recipient countries. However, it is not our task to expose any nefarious activities by government organisations at this stage, only to suggest that it is highly unlikely that condoms rise above this possibility!

Elsewhere, China recently purchased a manufacturing plant from Ansell-Americas in the USA, with help from the UN Fund for Population Activities, and Indonesia is to establish a factory in a joint venture with Japan's Sagami Rubber Industries. The International Planned Parenthood Federation doubled the number of condoms it distributed beteween 1978 and 1983 – from 280 million to 564 million – a sure sign of increasing awareness of the condom's value in developing countries.

'Social marketing' has a vital role to play in promoting this public awareness, using whatever means are available – TV, radio, newspapers and journals, posters, the cinema and theatre, displays, parades, competitions etc. There is little moralising about their use in developing countries, nor about their promotion, unlike most developed countries which still ban TV and radio advertising of

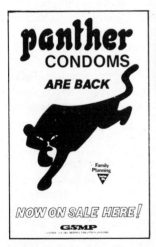 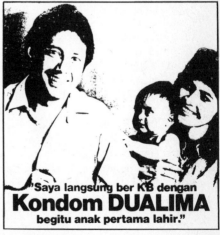

28. Two posters used in 'social marketing' promotions, the left from Ghana, where 200,000 condoms were sold in Accra during the first week of the campaign, and the right from Indonesia.

condoms, with the notable exceptions of Norway, Sweden, Denmark, Finland and Italy. Recently, for example, the *New York Times* and *Time* magazine refused to carry an AIDS-related condom advertisement featuring a woman saying 'I'll do a lot for love. But I'm not ready to die for it'. The major TV networks, NBC, ABC and CBS also at first refused to run the video version, but now two ABC affiliates have shown it and *Time* has reversed its policies – together with a number of US papers and magazines. Other TV advertisements are to follow, but the stations have restricted themselves to not promoting condoms as a method of birth control (as they have been on cable TV). Elsewhere, because of AIDS, Germany will see condoms promoted on television, and now that the law banning advertising them on French TV has been lifted, they will soon follow suit. Japan, too, even though AIDS has claimed so few lives and they are the world's largest consumers of condoms.

Major social marketing initiatives involving both public and private sectors have already been undertaken in Indonesia, Ghana and Mexico to respectively promote and sell custom-made 'Dualima', 'Panther' and 'Protektor' condoms. These are expected to be followed by similar projects in Panama, Liberia, Morocco and Brazil.

The picture in the USA is very similar to that in Britain. Although AIDS had officially surfaced there six or seven years ago, condom sales have fallen by half since 1976, until recently averaging 288 million condoms per year. Again, increasing public awareness, in spite of the lack of information from the Federal Government or the media, will doubtless guarantee a turnaround in the near future.

The US market is shared by two large manufacturers: Carter-Wallace Inc (which produces 'Trojans') takes approximately 56%, and Schmid (owned by none other than London International, producing 'Ramses' and 'Sheik') take 34%. Both companies make natural condoms, 'Naturalamb' and 'Fourex' respectively, using imported New Zealand lamb's intestines (no wonder none are made in Britain since it joined the EEC). The remaining 10% is split between Circle Rubber (a subsidy of Japan's Fuji Latex, and specialising in private-label products for others to market) and Ansell-Americas (owned by Australia's Pacific Dunlop, producing 'Life-Styles' and supplying the US military). A recent contender is Mentor Corporation who produce – at last – a condom specifically for women buyers (in the US women make up half the buyers of condoms), soon to be launched in Britain. Theirs is the only condom to offer anything out of the ordinary: an 'applicator hood' to help put it on, and an adhesive strip that prevents leaks and holds it in place.

US profits are considerable. This has enticed several new competitors to join the fray, both of whom will be importing Japanese condoms. Meanwhile a price war is about to break out amongst retailers – which in monetarist terms can only be a good thing: one New York drugstore chain plans to cut its condom prices by up to 30%. Given that the UK trails about four years behind the USA, maybe we will see a similar cut-price war between the supermarket chains and chemists in the near future, leaving LRC Products Ltd profitting as almost the sole supplier.

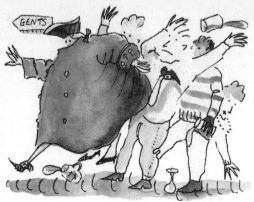

a desperate search . . .

The Condom in the World of Letters

I'll love thee much — Let me unseal the letter (King Lear)

We have already told you about Casanova, Madame de Sévigné, Pliny and other figures from the world of literature, showing how great minds have been occupied by condoms throughout history. Virgil, too, seems to refer not only to condoms, but to re-usable ones at that, saying of Hector that he 'redit exuvias indutus Achilli' (comes back wearing the armour stripped from Achilles). However, most real literary references to the condom in its early days are somewhat oblique, so that it is a great relief to come across a song which not only praises the condom, but also describes the material of which it is made and gives it an historical (tenth century) and geographical (strangely enough, Ireland!) setting:

> I was up to my ankles in turfmold
> At the peat contract down in the bog
> When me slinnie struck something hard, Sir:
> 'Twas a stick or a stone or a log.
>
> 'Twas a chest of the finest bog oak, Sir,
> And I wondered just what it might hide;
> So I chanced my luck with the fairies
> And I took just a wee peep inside.
>
> Now I know that you'll never believe me,
> 'Twas almost too good to be true,
> 'Twas an ancient old Irish French Letter,
> A relic of Brian Boru.

66

> Yes, an ancient old Irish French Letter
> Made of elk-hide and just one foot tall,
> With a wee golden tag at the end, Sir,
> With his name and his stud fees and all.
>
> And I cast my mind back through the ages,
> To the days of that hairy old Celt,
> Granwaille the Fair on the bed lay
> With Brian Boru in his pelt.
>
> And I heard him remark rather sternly,
> 'Now listen, we must get this right:
> You've had your own way for too long, dear,
> It's the hairy side outside tonight.'

This fascinating folk song, translated from the Irish, now only survives among those die-hard masochists, the members of the Rugby Football Union.

Ironically enough, in view of his later reputation *vis-á-vis* matters sexual, it was St Paul who seems first to have advocated the use of the sheath in his letter to the Ephesians (confirming, incidentally, the view of *Almonds for Parrots*, that the invention of the condom is to be ascribed to Divine Providence): 'Put on the whole armour of God, that you may be able to stand in the evil day, and having done all, to stand'. Had everyone followed his advice, there would have been no need for Dickens to write so regretfully: 'Accidents will happen, even in the best regulated families'.

The Eighteenth Century

Before the dark night of Victorian prudery set in, the condom was frequently celebrated in the literary world. *Almonds for Parrots* and *The Machine* were but two of these priapic works: who could disagree with sentiments like

> Happy the Man in whose close Pocket's found
> Whether with green or scarlet Ribbon bound
> A well-made CUNDUM . . .
> Great Ajax thus, the Grecian Chief, prepar'd,
> With seven-fold shield the Trojan Fury dar'd
> (. . .)
> With fresh found CUNDUM thou may'st swive each night
> Exstatic Harlot, and with fresh delight
> Unhurt, and satisfy thy best Desire. *(The Machine)*

Here we find Trojans mentioned two hundred years before their

appearance on the American market. Horace Walpole, who also
wrote Gothic Novels, writes in celebrating the birth of a daughter to
the Earl of Lincoln's mistress in 1743:

> You shall instruct her to remove the Fear.
> Nor but in Cundum arm'd, embrace her Dear.

In 1741, a gentleman by the (surely pseudonymous) name of Roger
Pheuquewell wrote *A New Description of Merryland* (a voyage
round the female anatomy, particularly the erogenous zones); in
the vagina:

> The climate is generaly warm, and sometimes so hot, that Strangers
> inconsiderately coming into it, have suffered exceedingly . . . But this
> dangerous Heat of the Climate, with all its dreadful Concomitants, is
> not so very terrible, but it may be guarded against by taking proper
> Precautions, and People might venture into it without much Hazard,
> even at the worst Seasons and in the most unhealthy Provinces; they
> need no more to avoid the Danger, but be careful always to wear
> *proper CLOTHING*, of which they have a sort that is very com-
> modious, and peculiarly adapted to this Country; it is made of an
> extraordinarily fine thin Substance, and contrived so as to be all of one
> Piece, and without a seam, only about the Bottom it is generally bound
> with a scarlet Ribbon for Ornament.

And, of course, though only recorded in Baroness Orczy's bowdler-
ised version of 1905, we have at the end of the century in the French
Revolution the rhyme recording the Scarlet Pimpernel's desperate
search for a condom:

> He seeks them here, he seeks them there,
> He seeks those Frenchies everywhere.

Vivat Victoria

Though she herself appeared on a condom, the atmosphere during
the good Queen's reign was not very conducive to the appearance of
condoms in literature. 'Walter', the author of the supposedly erotic,
but actually rather boringly pornographic *My Secret Life* wrote of
his use of French Letters in the 1880s: 'I gave Madeleine the
experience of a prick covered with a sheep's gut, but neither of us
liked it' and 'not liking the sensation – which cheats the pleasures of
both – I took my prick out, well greased the cundum outside, put it
on and up her again. We compared sensations, but both agreeing
that pleasure was largely lessened by the intervening skin . . . I took
it off.'

Fortunately, Norway comes to the rescue of the nineteenth century, with a book by Hans Jäger, which was published in Oslo (then still called Christiania) in 1885, the title of which was *Christiania Bohème*. It was translated into many languages, and regarded as a very good example of a macho book (then the order of the day). The book was immediately confiscated by the authorities, so the author re-issued it with the rather more innocent title *Christmas Stories*. But the Christmas stories had hardly hit the streets before they too were confiscated.

Why all the fuss? Was it because they had suddenly seen male chauvinism for whàt it was? Not a bit of it – the guardians of public morals accused the author of including 'indecent passages'. In fact, he mentioned condoms (which he called cordons: was this a cordon blue book?). One day when the laundress brought him his clean underwear, the hero of the book took a cordon from his pocket and said:

> 'Do you know what this is?'
> 'No,' said the laundress.
> 'Then I'll tell you: if you and I lie together, and I put on this thing' and as I said this, I unrolled the cordon so that she could see what it looked like, 'then it won't make a baby, because the stuff that makes babies stays in here' – and I stuck a finger into the cordon – 'and as you see, it doesn't let anything through, look' – and then I blew up the cordon – 'not even air gets through it.'
> She sat there, her face half turned away, and peeped at the cordon, but didn't say a word.
> 'Now,' I said, 'you can see, there's no reason to be afraid.
> (. . .)
> 'You're sitting here in my lap, and you like it when I caress you, and I like having you on my lap and caressing you; so we both want to sleep together, there's no danger, we won't be any the worse for it – you must admit it would be silly if we didn't use one of these cordons, wouldn't it?'
> She didn't answer, but went on peeping at the cordon, which now lay unrolled on the table.

Oh, Brave New World

With the dawn of the twentieth century, things changed radically. No history of the literary French Letter would be complete without James Joyce, of course, for sure enough, there in *Ulysses* we find 'two partly uncoiled rubber preservatives with reserve pockets, purchased by post from Box 32, P.O., Charing Cross, London, W.C.' (by which method Leopold Bloom had also purchased two 'erotic postcards'. To stay in Ireland, but advance a few decades, we find in J P Donleavy's *Ginger Man*:

I went into a chemist for those things when I first came to Ireland. I said, may I have a dozen. The man said to me, how dare you ask for such a thing and he hid behind the counter till I left. Naturally I thought he was mad. I went further up the street. Man with a great grin, how do and what not, I let my teeth out for a second. I noticed his were a little black. I put it to him pleasantly, asking for the American tips if possible. I saw his face go down, slouch of the jaw, hands twitch and a bottle break on the floor. The woman behind me indignantly swept out of the shop. The man in a hoarse whisper said he didn't deal in things like that. Also to please go away because the priest would put him out of business. I thought the gentleman must have something against the American tips which I prefer. I entered another shop and bought a bar of Imperial Leather for the class standing that was in it. Quietly I put it to him for a half dozen with English tips. I heard this man utter a low prayer, sweet mother of Jesus, save us from the licentious. He then blessed himself and opened the door for me to leave. I left thinking Ireland a most peculiar country.

In England, in the thirties, both Orwell and Huxley get in on the act, Orwell in *Keep the Aspidistra Flying*, where his hero, Gordon Comstock (an apt name in the circumstances), sees the condom as a symbol of the economic and social collapse that has followed the First World War:

'You can see our whole civilisation written there. The imbecility, the emptiness, the desolation! You can't look at it without thinking of French Letters and machine guns.'

And, failed poet that he is, he includes it in his 'London Pleasures', referring to the

'Money-god . . . who . . . lays the sleek estranging shield
Between the lover and his bride.

and Huxley in *Brave New World*, where

round her waist she wore a silver-mounted green morocco-surrogate cartridge belt, bulging with the regulation supply of contraceptives . . .
　　'Perfect!' cried Fanny enthusiastically . . . 'And what a perfectly *sweet* Malthusian belt!'

It's not entirely clear that the contraceptives meant are condoms, but the image of the condom replacing the cartridge is too pleasing to be missed. Make love not war, with a vengeance!

In the fifties and sixties Britain, the campus novel and the Northern realist novel were in vogue, and it's no surprise to find condoms rearing their head once again in this context. Victor, in

Stan Barstow's *A Kind of Loving*, has problems about getting hold of them:

> 'Willy, when you get yourself fixed up with a bird – you know, on a sure thing – where do you get your tackle from?'
> (. . .)
> 'Where do you get fixed up? Have you any on you now?'
> ''Smatter of fact I'm right out at the moment. But you can buy 'em. Just walk into a shop and ask for 'em.'
> 'Which shop?'
> 'Oh, any chemist's. Doesn't your barber flog 'em?'
> 'I don't know.'
> 'A lot of 'em do.'
> 'Anyway, my barber's a pal of the Old Feller's.'
> 'Well, there's plenty o' places.'
> 'Suppose you go into a chemist's and a bird comes to serve you?'
> 'So what? She knows just what they're for just like anybody else.'
> 'I couldn't ask a bird, Willy. I'd be embarrassed.'

This scene is transposed in the film to one in which Alan Bates enters a chemist's shop, is met by a formidable woman assistant, and comes out with a bottle of 'Lucozade'. His next meeting with Ingrid, his girl, then goes as follows:

> 'Did you get anything . . . you know . . . ?' she says.
> 'No. I went downtown on Saturday but I couldn't bring meself to go into a shop an' ask.'
> 'We'd better not . . . you know . . . go so far then, had we?'

But of course they do, with predictable results. The Catholic characters in David Lodge's novels have sin and guilt to contend with as well: the protagonist in *The British Museum is Falling Down*, having produced a child almost every year of his marriage, in spite of contortions with thermometers every day by his wife in an attempt to work out her 'safe' period, determines to buy some of the offending articles (though actually in order to commit adultery). He is about to enter a famous 'Surgical Store' on the Edgeware Road, when out of the mist looms his parish priest (an Irishman, of course), who enters with him, delivers a lecture on the evils of contraception, and foils our hero's nefarious intentions. Lodge it is who is responsible for a poem about the sheath, which includes the lines:

> The rubber gloves of prudent lechery
> Leave no traces
> Rifling the virgin's bottom drawer.

His fellow-academic Malcolm Bradbury's Professor Treece, in *Eating People is Wrong*, finds himself in an embarrassing situation at the University's Christmas Ball:

> From behind, someone tapped him on the shoulder. It was Oliver. 'Do you happen to have any contraceptives on you?' he asked confidentially.
> Merrick promptly opened up his wallet and went carefully through it. Should be able to oblige, old boy,' he said.
> 'Good,' said Oliver. 'Always wanted to do it outside, you know, ever since I read *Sons and Lovers*.'
> 'No, sorry, old boy, I'm out,' said Merrick. 'I didn't think I'd be coming tonight.'
> Treece took out his wallet and looked in it; if he hadn't been drunk he would have been shocked, and if he hadn't been drunk he wouldn't have tried to pretend he had any, when he most certainly hadn't.
> 'Don't let me take your last,' said Oliver.
> 'Sorry, I havent', said Treece, slapping his wallet to.
>   'Just have to risk it,' said Oliver, departing.

What else happens to all the condoms that keep popping up in this modern literature?

Guess, dear Readers!

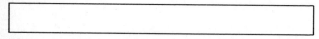

Answers to be filled in here please

Now read what follows, and find out if you were right. Probably not, although our first example is something that rarely if ever happens:

> 'I'm sorry,' said the purser, and pursed his lips, as if he'd found a French Letter in the salad. (Jon Michelet, Norway)

Other people don't toss their condoms in the salad, but into the water, to the delight of fishermen and women:

> Ingri was a character. She had a collection of forty condoms. We used to fish them out by the bridge, where the river flowed very slowly because of all the chocolate wrappers and dead fish. (Merethe Lindström, Norway)

Yet others give them away:

> Just look at this super balloon, it's like a   warf with a sack on its back when you blow it up properly. I don't know if it can be used for something more essential, the lady in the shop didn't understand when I tried to ask her. (Bergljot Hobäk Haff, Norway)

Norwegians, of course, are not the only ones to write about condoms. Americans, too, have had their say. Take Alex Portnoy, for
example, as neurotically and hypochondriacally afraid of the
slightest danger as any American tourist. When a friend persuades
his girlfriend to do young Alex a favour, everything is fine – or is it:

> Now I have absolutely nothing to worry about except the Trojan I have
> been carrying around so long in my wallet that inside its tinfoil wrapper
> it has probably been half eaten away by mold. One spurt and the whole
> thing will go flying in pieces all over the inside of Bubbles Giardi's box –
> and *then* what do I do?
> To be sure that these Trojans really hold up under pressure, I have
> been down in my cellar all week filling them with quart after quart of
> water – expensive as it is, I have been using them to jerk off into, to see
> if they will stand up under simulated fucking conditions. So far so good.
> Only what about the sacred one that has by now left an indelible
> imprint of its shape on my wallet, the very special one I have been
> saving to get laid with, with the lubricated tip? How can I possibly
> expect no damage to have been done after sitting on it in school –
> crushing it in that wallet – for nearly six months?

First sexual experiences seem so often to be bound up with condoms
(or the lack of them!). Lisa Alther's heroine in *Kinflicks* has one of
the most alien:

> He turned out the overhead light, throwing the room into blackness.
> I heard the sound of a zipper being unzipped nearby. Then I heard a
> tearing sound, followed by a snapping sound. My eyes wide open in the
> blackness, I saw something coming at me. It was the size and shape of a
> small salami, lime green and glowing fluorescently. Small green
> prongs, like on a space satellite, protruded from the rounded end. As I
> watched with the absorption of St Theresa viewing the stigmata, this
> phosphorescent vision descended until it was hovering over my abdo-
> men. Then, as I watched, the object plunged itself between my legs. I
> felt it entering me with a searing pain.
> (. . .)
> Finally, as I was mentally drumming my fingers on the platform,
> Clem stopped abruptly. The lime salami reemerged and floated in the
> air for a few moments, looking as though it were about to ascend into
> the heavens, whence it had come. Then there was a snapping noise and
> it vanished.
> (. . .)
> Our second attempt wasn't much more impressive than the first. By
> the lantern light he donned an orange neon condom whose foil wrapper
> read 'Fiesta Brand'. 'Where do you get those?' I asked nonchalantly.
> Joe Bob's Dixie Delight condoms had been a utilitarian tan. Perhaps
> that was why I had never let him screw me. Could condoms, like Holy
> Communion, be an outward and visible sign of one's inward and
> spiritual grace?

'Floyd gets 'em somewhere. He says that French tickler like I used last time drives Maxine Pruitt wild.'

'Oh yeah?' What was wrong with me that I hadn't been driven wild too? If I was to be driven wild at some point in the future, would I *know* that I was being driven wild?

Back in Britain, we have the other side of the coin in Brian Aldiss's *Hand-Reared Boy:*

The baby problem could be overcome, at least in theory, by using French Letters. But French Letters had to be bought. It was not just the cash. It was stepping into the little barber's at the end of Chapel Road and actually asking for a packet for a friend. The only time I dared to go in was one day when I thought I was on a sure thing for the evening, a rather plump girl, called, so help her, Esmeralda, who belonged to the tennis club I did. I spent about an hour of indecision, riding past the barber's shop and round the corner on my bike, at various speeds. Finally I did go in and buy a packet of three Frenchies.
(. . .)
'You can have a look. That won't hurt either of us. But I may as well tell you now, *love*, that you aren't going to get anything more than a look.'
'The sight of it may drive me mad!'
'That's up to you, not me!'
I patted my pocket. 'You don't have to be frightened. I've brought some things.
This announcement did frighten her. She saw I meant business. The trouble was, I was also frightened, and didn't know whether or not I meant business. I had never worn a French Letter.
(. . .)
But I could feel my hard-on going soft. I extracted it from my flies and started fumbling with the French Letter packet. I got one out, pushing the other two back into my pocket. I balanced it on my glans penis and begin awkwardly to try to roll it down. Esmeralda had been laying back in a languorous posture. She sat up and watched with interest.
I got the damned thing on, wrinkled and repulsive.
(. . .)
We were both nervous. It would not go in.
I did not know where to put my penis in that chubby pink pocket. I didn't know enough about female anatomy. I had never explored my sister. I pushed and sweated, and the damned French Letter meant I could not feel her pleasant parts.
'You're hurting me love. I'm a virgin – I think you'd better give over.'
Did she invoke the middle-class spectre of virginity to save my face? I don't know. But I was glad enough to desist, and pulled the French Letter off in exasperation.

Horace Stubbs, for such is our hero's name, is a little luckier in the forces in the Far East during the War (reported in the sequel, *A Soldier Erect*):

> I could hear myself groaning while the hag by the bedside was trying to get two rupees off me for a French Letter. Cursing, I gave her two half-rupee pieces and told her to fuck off.
> The girl's body was slightly oily. She was co-operating now . . . She peeled the French Letter on to my weapon in a prosaic housewifely manner while I – in what animal past was I, tunneling through a dense familiar element, triumphant, cock-a-hoop?
> (. . .)
> This girl wrapped her legs round me like a stone-age lass, and pummelled me with her heels on my bum as I shot my roe with considerable force and splendour into what was probably a secondhand French Letter.

Apart from the invention of a brand of condom named 'Sheikh' after Rudolf Valentino's triumph, one of the best US condom stories comes from Lillian Hellman's time as a script-writer. The film star Harry C. Potter (who?) was being a bit of a pain to her and one of her colleagues, and so they decided to get their own back on him. In those days you could get match books with pictures of film stars on them, so they bought a job-lot of them. They wanted to put a French Letter inscribed with 'Best Wishes from Harry C. Potter' in each of them and spread them around unobtrusively at a cocktail party they were planning. This was forty years ago, and printing technology wasn't as advanced as it is now, so the two conspirators tried to use wax which they melted on a stove to make the letters (the writing, not the condoms). And that's where their problem started: cold wax wouldn't stay on, hot wax burnt holes on the condoms. 'After a while the condoms in the drugstore were sold out, and one of the moments which stays most clearly in my memory is the salesman staring at George when he asked for another dozen boxes.' And it took another two weeks before the problem was solved. They didn't do any other work, importunate producers were fobbed off with very thin excuses, but the result of it all was: 27 condoms with a bright green inscription: 'Best Wishes from Harry C. Potter'. So Lillian Helman and her colleague went off and got drunk, as any sensible person in their shoes would have done.

But when they'd slept off the hangover, they realised their troubles weren't over yet: they still had to roll up the condoms to stick them in the match books, but the condoms wouldn't play ball. Either they were thicker than they are nowadays, or the match books were smaller. But then a very uptight and prim secretary solved the problem in two shakes of a duck's tail: the condoms needed to be folded first lengthways and then sideways, and then they fitted into the match books.

And what happened then? Not a whiff of scandal! No one mentioned the condoms, and in their annoyance Lillian Hellman and her colleague never said a word about them, then or later.

Flannelled Fools and Muddied Oafs

One of the last bastions of male chauvinism is the sports' field, where outdated and old-fashioned modes of behaviour still survive. A few examples from this seamier side of our men's past, just kept alive in drunken song, will have to suffice – if just to remind us what they should forget! Perhaps the most famous of all is *Eskimo Nell*, who comes from the Far North where

> The nights are sixty below,
> Where it's so damn' cold
> That the Johnnies are sold
> Wrapped up in a ball of snow.

Old fertility rites are found in *The Ball of Kirriemuir*, yet even here, amid all the dionysiac revelry, the vicar's wife is to be found 'sitting by the fire, knitting rubber Johnnies from an India rubber tyre'. Further back:

> In days of old, when knights were bold
> And Johnnies weren't invented,
> They'd wrap a sock about their cock
> And babies were prevented.

There are family sagas:

> My Grandad sells cheap prophylactics
> And punctures the teats with a pin,
> For Grandma gets rich from abortions,
> My God, how the money rolls in.

And to show the classlessness of the condom, even the world of upper-class public schools for girls features:

> Our sports mistress she is the best,
> She teaches us to develop our chest,
> So we wear tight sweaters
> And carry French Letters
> For we are from Roedean School.

Finally, there is a poignant song to the tune of *Home on the Range*, lamenting the dangers of contraceptive carelessness:

> Torn, torn at the end,
> His '█████' was torn at the end;
> He wouldn't have been
> If his father had seen
> That his '█████' was torn at the end.

The limerick, too, often celebrates the condom: here one example must represent the many:

> There was a schoolmarm of Devizes
> Who was done at the local assizes
> For teaching young boys
> Matrimonial joys
> And giving French Letters as prizes.

And Now, the Eighties

In 1986, three books appeared in paperback which are germane to our theme. Rather like the opening of a joke, there was an American, a Czech and an Englishwoman. First, we have Wendy Perriam with *The Stillness, the Dancing*. The heroine's daughter has an affair with a Frenchman while on holiday, and then returns to her boyfriend at home:

> 'Hey, come *out!*'
> He almost didn't. She loved that, too. The danger, the excitement . . . She only worried afterwards, especially if her period was late. Martin promised it was safe . . . Pierre had used a '█████' – or whatever the French equivalent was – a decadent looking black one. She was almost disappointed when he came inside her . . . With Pierre she hadn't seen it at all, just a limp black chrysalis with something white and sticky at the bottom. He had left it behind in the attic and she had worried someone would find it in the morning, but what could she have done with it – put it in her handbag?

In an earlier novel of hers, *Born of Woman*, there is an episode which shows just how in this, as in other fields, history repeats itself:

> He couldn't screw her, anyway – not even conventional fashion. It wasn't just the funeral – he had no '█████' with him. He had never entered Jennifer in a whole three years of marriage without that rubber skin between them. He hated '█████' – damn-fool fiddly things. But Jennifer refused the Pill, rejected every contraceptive. Jennifer wanted babies. Well, so did he – not just *yet*, that's all . . . Anyway, even without the babies, he preferred to put a barrier between himself and any woman, including his own wife. It was safer, somehow, cleaner. Stopped him touching her most private places. It meant he could keep a

shell around himself, one last barrier – enter her and yet still be separate. Hester [his mother] would have approved of '███████' if she had permitted sex at all.

But he finds a back way round his problem – using a form of contraception widely practised in Africa.

The Czech is Josef Skvorecky, and in his novel *The Engineer of Human Souls* he interweaves the present of a character not too different from himself, a professor at a Canadian University, with the past in wartime and postwar Czechoslovakia. As a professor, he visits Paris with one of his students:

> Irene pulled her toys out of the suitcase with the breathless enthusiasm of youth. When we arrived at Yvette's Hotel on the Place Convention, and found ourselves alone in a beautiful Parisian *fille-de-joie* chamber with a wide double bed and a bidet hiding behind a folding screen, she produced a package she had smuggled into the land of love from the Lovecraft shop in Toronto. It contained twelve condoms. Now I stand looking at those apostles of natural vice, spread out on the non-connubial bed, and the disgusting rubber proturberances on them make me feel slightly ill.
>
> 'Ugh, Irene!' I say to the girl standing modestly beside this display in an elegant dress bought especially for Paris, entirely convinced that she has made me a gift of unconventional delight. 'What are they?'
>
> 'Safes'.
>
> 'I thought they were special educational models to demonstrate what malignant tumours look like.'

And thirdly, from America, there is John Irving's *Cider House Rules*. Homer Wells was born in an orphanage, but goes to live on an apple farm:

> He even liked Herb Fowler. He'd been with Herb less than two minutes when the prophylactic sailed his way and struck him in the forehead. All Meany Hyde had said was, 'Hi, Herb. This here is Homer Wells – he's Wally's pal from Saint Cloud's.' And Herb had flipped the rubber at Homer.
>
> 'Wouldn't be so many orphans if more people put these on their joints,' Herb said.
>
> Homer Wells had never seen a prophylactic in a commercial wrapper. The ones that Dr. Larch kept at the hospital, and distributed to so many of the women, in handfuls, were sealed in something plain and see-through, like wax paper; no brand names adorned them. Dr Larch was always complaining that he didn't know where all the rubbers were going, but Homer knew that Melony had helped herself on many occasions. It had been Melony, of course, who had introduced Homer to prophylactics.

And during Thanksgiving at the orphanage:

> In lieu of balloons, Dr Larch distributed prophylactics to Nurse Angela
> and Nurse Edna, who – despite their distaste for the job – inflated the
> rubbers and dipped them in bowls of green and red food coloring.
> When the coloring dried, Mrs Grogan painted the orphans' names on
> the rubbers, and Homer and Candy hid the brightly colored prophlac-
> tics all over the orphanage.
> 'It's a rubber hunt,' said Wilbur Larch. 'We should have saved the
> idea up for Easter. Eggs are expensive.'

Something Completely Different

No consideration of the role of the condom in literature would be
complete without mentioning the works of Tom Sharpe, who
deserves, if anyone ever did, the title of Doctor of (French) Letters.
It would take a work of much larger scope to give details of all the
many and varied condoms and uses made of them that appear in his
novels – some diligent scholar might take it as a research topic so
we'll confine ourselves to a few of the more striking examples. In
Wilt, Gaskell and Sally Pringsheim are stuck in a boat which has
broken down in the Norfolk Broads:

> 'You got those rubbers you use?' he asked suddenly.
> 'Jesus, at a time like this you get a hard on,' said Sally, 'Forget sex.
> Think of some way of getting us off here.'
> 'I have,' said Gaskell, 'I want those skins!'
> 'You going to float downriver on a pontoon of condoms?'
> 'Balloons,' said Gaskell. 'We blow them up and paint letters on them
> and float them in the wind . . .'
> 'Where's your nail varnish?' Gaskell asked when he had finished and
> twelve contraceptives littered the cabin . . .
> Gaskell came out on deck with the contraceptives. He had tied them
> together and painted on each one a single letter with nail varnish so that
> the whole read HELP SOS HELP. He climbed up on the cabin roof
> and launched them into the air. They floated up for a moment, were
> caught in the light breeze and sagged down into the water.

Not only do they not fly, the message doesn't remain clear either,
and the condoms produce a whole series of senseless anagrams,
much to the surprise of the local and somewhat alcoholic vicar:

> . . . he was startled to see something wobbling above the reeds on Eel
> Stretch. It looked like balloons, white sausage-shaped balloons that
> rose briefly and disappeared . . . If he was right, and he didn't know
> whether he wanted to be or not, the morning was being profaned by a
> cluster of contraceptives, inflated contraceptives, wobbling erratically

where by the nature of things no contraceptive had ever wobbled before. At least he hoped it was a cluster. He was so used to seeing things in twos when they were in fact ones that he couldn't be sure if what looked like a cluster of inflated contraceptives wasn't just one or better still none at all.

Condoms also form a major theme in *Porterhouse Blue;* Zipser, a research student at the Cambridge College of the title, falls in love with his bedmaker, and decides to equip himself for the fray. After a series of attempts (including not one but several haircuts) to buy French Letters in the normal way, he ends up with two cartons, containing a gross each. Now he has the problem of disposing of them – which, as we all know, isn't easy. They won't flush, the quantity is immense, so eventually he fills them with gas and sticks them up the chimney in his room. Some escape, but the cold outside makes them descend, causing an embarrassing exhibition in the college quad: and poor Zipser himself is hoist with his own petard when his bedmaker lights the gas fire in his room, just as they are about to consummate their passion. The subsequent explosion not only brings about the demise of both student and bedmaker, but also blows down a considerable part of the building they are in. Other characters in his novels are involved in various trials of this kind, but pride of place, and the grand climax of our literary section must go to *The Throwback.* For reasons we needn't go into, a condom is lubricated with something other than spermicide, with the following results:

> What was in the French Letter that Colonel Finch-Potter nudged over his penis at half past eight the following night had certainly kept. He was vaguely aware that the contraceptive felt more slippery than usual when he took it out of the box but the full effect of the oven cleaner made itself felt when he had got it three-quarters on and was nursing the rubber ring right down to achieve maximum protection from syphilis. The next moment all fear of contagious disease had fled his mind and far from trying to get the thing on he was struggling to get the fucking thing off as quickly as possible and before irremediable damage had been done. He was unsuccessful. Not only was the contraceptive slippery but the oven cleaner was living up to its maker's claim to be able to remove grease baked on to the interior of a stove like lightning. With a scream of agony Colonel Finch-Potter gave up his manual attempts to get the contraceptive off before what felt like galloping leprosy took its fearful toll and dashed towards the bathroom in search of a pair of scissors . . . Colonel Finch-Potter's howls had long since ceased. He lay on the kitchen floor with a cheese-grater and worked assiduously and with consummate courage on the thing that had been his penis. That the corrosive contraceptive had long since disintegrated under the striations of the breadknife he neither knew nor cared. It was

sufficient to know that the rubber ring remained and that his penis had swollen to three times its normal size. It was in an insane effort to grate it down from a phallic gargoyle to something more precise that the colonel worked.

And with that salutory thought, we leave the world of letters and move on to condoms themselves, which like flowers are very colourful and varied.

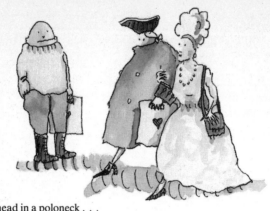

a skinhead in a poloneck . . .

You and Your Condom

You're never alone using a condom! Just think that over 40 million couples all over the world are relying on them too, supplied with a stock of some 5,000 million condoms produced by over twenty factories worldwide. Although in the UK we cannot possibly hope to compete with the staggering 25% of this total that the Japanese consume, or indeed the 20% slice the Chinese claim, UK condom sales are on the increase. According to a survey conducted by Mintel Publications in November 1985 (Market Intelligence), the 20 million pounds we spent that year on some 115 million items of slippery latex was an increase of 15% on figures for the previous five years. And despite the condom's low personal preference amongst most of the men we know, it is now the second most popular form of contraception in the UK, only pipped to the post, according to the Family Planning Association's hit list, by the Pill.

Still, there's a lot of difference between driving a Renault 4 and a Rolls Royce so it's absolutely imperative for men and women to know their way around the market. There's nothing quite as embarrassing as dressing down when you should be dressing up, and with the wide choice of condoms it is quite possible to find something to suit almost every occasion. There are pink condoms and green condoms, patterned condoms, condoms with horns, delay reaction condoms, short and long condoms, rough and smooth condoms to court your pleasure. But remember the well-known maxim 'It ain't the meat, it's the motion' before you make your purchase, because not all of them will enhance your individual performance.

And for those who enjoy statistics, and would like to know how seven different condoms compared with each other, see the Appendix (in this book!).

A Question of Size

In the good old days when condoms were re-usable, LRC made three sizes; small, medium and large. No prizes for guessing which size proved the least popular. These days condoms all seem to be a uniform size in the UK. LRC however do acknowledge that not all nations boast such large attributes as the UK man. They make condoms in two sizes, Occidental (for the big boys in the UK) and Oriental for the smaller versions in far flung continents. French condom maunfacturers make their condoms 3cms larger than the UK varieties! All over the world it appears that condoms are rebuffed on size. When the Americans first started exporting condoms to Thailand, they were far too big. As popular folklore has it, the Thais were forced to tie string around their condoms and then around their waists to secure the items in place, but then what would you expect to do in a place called Thailand?

In 1985 the Swedes sent 10 million condoms to Kenya. They were immediately returned – the Swedish outsize condom was an inch and half too short for the Kenyans. The Australians also sent back a consignment imported from Asia as too small. Mind you, these will probably find themselves in the capable hands of a company like Aegis Ltd (one of the large mail-order condom organisations in the UK). They certainly don't let anything as insignificant as size interfere with a good thing. They just market the smaller brands of condoms as 'Snug Fits' and have nothing but praise from their grateful clients. Their 'Big Boy' condoms sell like hot cakes, too.

But now a run down of the more popular and easily purchased varieties on the UK market. Remember, over the counter purchases tend to be about as inspiring as selecting 'American Tan' tights in supermarkets. You may need to resort to discreet mail order, or to some of London's more seedier sex venues (the latter not recommended pricewise). For the gay market prospects are slightly rosier. Specialist gay outlets in London cater not for the pervert you are often assumed to be in a heterosexual sex shop, but as a responsible individual with a normal sex drive and seeking an alternative from the mundane.

Flesh Tones versus Black Condoms

Ten to one if you think of a condom it will either be pink, cream or beige, subtle colours which denote subtle sex. These staid clinical hues are what the rest of the world associates with the British Condom. No frills or picadils, no exotic connotations – they're practical no-nonsense items. The most popular UK colour for condoms is coral (LRC favour this delicate skintone for the majority of their products). Even behind the most promising packaging, like the plastic capsule containers dispensed by some vending machines, there lurks an uninspiring putty-coloured condom. These condoms which we hold so dear to our heart are not as well received in other parts of the globe; in Scandinavia, they are the pits, and the least favoured colour of all.

Interestingly, it is black condoms which are especially popular in Scandinavia and with the gay community in the UK, although it's hard to say why, unless the myth of the sexual prowess of black men has some connection (one participant in Journeyman's survey actually noted that black condoms turned him on). Coal black until it's unfurled, it quickly turns to an uninspiring slate grey, at which point any association with suckable liquorice vanishes. One advantage is that it does make the penis invisible in the dark and it is impossible to see what is being placed into it, large, small, broad, flat or round. It also has advantages for day time use since it makes a nice contrast with the milky white skin so common in Nothern and Western Europe. Any evidence that blacks use these devices in preference to antiseptic pink or buff is not forthcoming, but one can assume that anyone not wishing to draw attention to their penis by adding a technicolour hue might well prefer to linger in the shadow of a black condom. It is quite likely that those Caucasians who prefer black condoms are more aware of their appearance than those who opt for pastels. Here, then, is a useful tip for women to watch out for; gross vanity, as we all know, can affect performance.

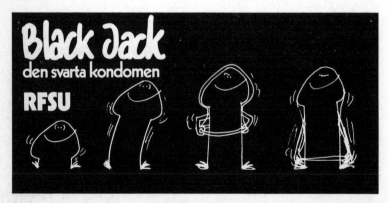

29. Swedish 'Black Jack' promotion, imitated elsewhere in the world. Treating the condom in this way avoids the moral dilemma of showing men sexually aroused!

You can buy black condoms over the counter in chemists now that they are one of the more daring items made by LRC, but there are alternatives marketed by other companies.

Assault-course Condoms

Many condoms come replete with added features these days. Some boast lines down their length, some lines around their width, some have what look like outcrops of 'zits', some enormous warts, and some like Japanese varieties are wrinkled all over. All of course are designed to increase the sexual pleasure of the woman, and any that succeed will do so by auto-suggestion rather than physically, as the whole concept is a myth – still, whatever turns you on. Of course, any increase in sexual pleasure experienced by the man will also be in the mind, unless he turns his condom inside out and survives the ordeal. These condoms all have names of epic proportions: 'Deadly Nightshafts', 'Rough Riders', 'Rugged' and 'Wrinklers', or names that imply satisfaction for the woman eg 'Stimula' and 'Arouser'. Women should not however be frightened by these devices, for as uncomfortable as they sound they are all quite tame, as a friend of ours discovered. She assumed that a ribbed condom would bear a striking resemblance to corrugated iron, but was disappointed by its subtle profile.

But take note, not everything condom-shaped serves the same purpose. Novelty condoms (or 'carnival condoms' as Anja Meulenbelt, a Dutch feminist, has called them) may come with Mickey Mouse heads, elephant heads, and assorted cactii-like tips, but they are not contraceptives and not prophylactics either. These thick,

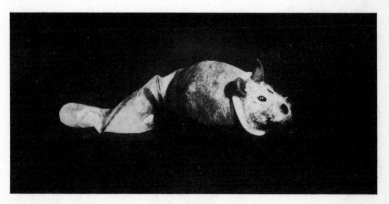

30. A condom tailpiece? A Mickey Mouse condom? Send your suggestions to Journeyman – but don't expect any prizes.

lurid, latex condoms have generous holes and flaws and need to be worn with a regular condom liner, advice often missing from the packaging. Basically they are toys and should be viewed as such. But a word of warning to the women/men on the receiving end of horned 'ticklers' – some have sharp and potentially dangerous thick rubber outcrops, literally welded to the latex. These are quite capable of causing toxic shock system (in women), or at least scratching delicate internal surfaces and we don't recommend their use.

Venereal Variations

If you are looking for a totally constricting experience, try 'Snug Fit'. These are small, skin-tight condoms, said by some to increase arousal and by others to stop the circulation. These wouldn't remotely interest the buyers of 'Big Boy' condoms but, be warned, men that opt for these extra big condoms, are not normally the types that have the where-with-all to fill them! For minimal coverage but maximum staying power try American Tips, the shortest condoms on the market. Made popular by the American forces during the war, these condoms have a habit of getting lost in action and can lead to all sorts of interesting bedtime manoeuvres. An American Tip is literally a cap that makes contact with your flesh about a third of the way up the penis and held in position by an extremely tight rubber ring. More often than not the American Tip has more staying power than the man who's suffering it, *and that* is why you will often find the 'grin and bear it' type wearing one.

Passion Killers

We are not talking here about winceyette nighties and cold cream, we're talking about how to control men's unbridled passion and get a better deal in bed for ourselves. There's a wonder substance called Benzocaine, which really does prove to be a girl's best friend. Benzocaine is a numbing agent, a local (very mild) anaesthetic, and a small splodge at the tip of a condom won't send your partner's penis to sleep, but it will give you a chance to get what you want. Totally harmless, most condoms with names like 'Honeymoon' 'Prolong' or 'Personal Ritardante' are spiked with the said substance. The results of Journeyman's survey certainly prove its effectiveness: in the case of the one tested, it was considered 21% above average at prolonging intercourse. Just one note of caution though, make sure it is on the right way round or it will backfire on you. If you are not sure what sort of condom to use, try 'Triple Action'. This one has everything – it's specially contoured, ribbed for extra stimulation and has a built-in delayer to keep you going. Definitely a condom that ensures total confusion: it will have you wondering whether you're coming, going or gone!

Tutti Frutti

'Lurid Lime', 'Strawberry Slurp' and 'Bold Banana' are just three of the many fruit-flavoured condoms designed to get you salivating. These condoms not only smell like a fruit salad they taste like one too. Whether you opt for them depends very much on whether you like the taste and smell of latex mingled with lime/strawberry/apple/ orange etc. Or perhaps association with the forbidden fruits may enhance their attraction! The sort of men that gravitate towards fruity condoms tend to be nature lovers, members of the Ecology Party, lovers of – and in – the great outdoors. The Scandinavians and the Germans have a preference for a fresh apple variation on the theme. Indeed, in a poll carried out in Hamburg with 34 male members of the city's alternative party a staggering 33.7% revealed a preference for apple-flavoured condoms. One wonders whether they also had a preference for girls called Eve! Journeyman's survey seemed to indicate some confusion among the British. 11% couldn't tell which flavour they had been sent, and another 15% got it wrong. Still, this didn't prevent them from being a more enjoyable experience – over half thought they measured up to expectations.

Party Colours

Yes, you can show your political allegiance in these. Red, green, and blue are available, but we recommend that you buy a reputable brand because coloured condoms are not reknown for being colour-fast. They are also not generally as safe as the conservative pink and buffs. The least safe colour is green which, according to a report in the Australian consumer magazine *Choice* (1982), had a failure rate bad enough to make you turn that exact same shade. The colour they were talking about was a dark green condom and one of a selection from a '█████' coloured pack they tested. However, you can rest assured that even these dark green condoms will not run; LRC has at least perfected that technique. The world is indeed a fickle place when it comes to colour choice – the Kenyans like red, the Japanese like black and baby blue, and in Egypt, Thailand, Jamaica and warmer, more relaxed climes, they literally party it up with blues, greens, pinks and yellows.

Back-to-Nature Condoms

Vegans or vegetarians should stop reading here . . . These natural membrane condoms, made from lamb's intestines, are strictly for carnivores and, like all gastronomic delicacies, come pickled in an aspic-like jelly. 'Skins' as they are often called, are the Rolls Royce of condoms and cost twice the price of humble latex. Devotees claim they increase sensitivity, and don't cling as tight as latex. The natural lubricant is thought to stimulate vaginal secretions and, as these condoms transmit bodyheat more easily, hotter sex. You can also look forward to unwrapping something that looks like a well-chewed piece of gum, dripping jelly with a smell not of latex, but something far worse.

the Rolls Royce of condoms . . .

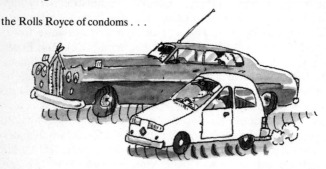

Popular in Western Europe and with a following in the USA, skins are a fairly rare commodity here. Natural lamb condoms are imported from the USA and are usually available by mail order but, be warned, they don't go through the same rigorous testing as their latex brothers. Purists may like to note that Casanova himself donned a very similar item and perhaps decorated them with ribbons, to distract his conquests from the unusual smell.

Safety-first Condoms

History comes full circle with the influx of newstyle condoms. The new strain of extra durable and all-encompassing condoms now available are not for the prevention of babies, but for the very same reason that Casanova wore them, to prevent the spread of STDs. And not just the old favourites like syphilis and gonorrhoea, but the new incurables diseases like Herpes and the killer AIDS.

First, the delectable 'Anti VD' sheath. Now this really is the condom that comes closest to the raincoat. Generously cut, this sheath is all enveloping; it not only runs the length of the penis, but it also covers the testicles as well. It certainly reaches the parts the other condoms don't reach, and prevents a larger part of the anatomy coming into contact with anything unpleasant. The main problem with this hefty piece of apparatus is the strong elastication at the top of the scrotum which holds it in place, and plays hell with the pubic hair. One gay guy we spoke to, who once used the device, said his partner initially mistook his shrieks for ecstasy rather than agony, but not for long, the clamping action of the 'Anti VD' sheath soon made any form of sex impossible. These sheaths are milky white, come folded, rather than sealed in discreet packets, and make huge bulges in breast pockets. Rubber fetishists probably have a field day with them, but they certainly need lubrication.

The other armour-plated device currently on sale is the Pro-phyltex 'Red Stripe' brand imported from France. Initially sold into the gay market, they come complete with a handy leaflet about where you can put it and where you can't. They are a buff trans-parent latex, and so highly lubricated they make your fingers slip off the typewriter keys. They are also huge compared to a regular condom (is this telling us something we didn't know about the gay man?). But their main selling point is their strength; they are far better equipped for anal intercourse, and less lightly to tear than thinner condoms. Gays may also prefer this heavyweight condom aesthetically, because it has a rounded end rather than a teat, and therefore makes a far more appealing silhouette (interestingly, Journeyman's survey suggests this may also be true of heterosexuals as well: on appearance alone they were rated 17% above average). As yet these condoms are not available in the favourite gay colour – black.

A third contender, Soplex Ltd, arrived on the scene in January 1987 with their 'Knight Barrier' condom. The freshest latex condom around (straight from the tree to the Malaysian factory production line makes for a better product, says Soplex). Well, this is certainly a heavyweight condom: 0.09mm thick compared to the average 0.06–0.07mm of UK products (the opposite extreme is a Japanese import at 0.03mm). Milky white, lubricated, and with one added feature – it's been made smaller to offer the firmest fit and therefore added security. As Soplex are wholesalers rather than retailers, watch out for this condom popping up in all manner of disguises.

You can also buy condoms that have an additional feature, a built-in spermicide. There are no tests to prove whether these are any more effective than untreated condoms, but they are recom-mended as nerve soothers for the insecure. Using a spermicide increases the effectiveness of the condom, and chemicals like nonoxynol-9, present in several widely-used spermicides, de-activates the AIDS virus.

Self-adhesive Condoms

The latest in condom technology, a veritable rubber revelation, this condom's secret weapon is a half-inch strip of medical grade adhesive towards the end of the shaft which bonds your Johnny into position. And very sensible, too (apparently 1 in 10 condoms come off in action). UK trial tests carried out at St Mary's Hospital in Paddington have been encouraging. It has been found less likely to tear (it moves with you and not against you), it is less likely to leak (the sperm are all trapped up the pointed end), it clings tight even on the most flacid penis and is well suited for anal sex.

As you can imagine, it's very important to put this condom on the right way round or a one-night stand could develop into a very binding relationship. For these purposes this clever all-rounder comes complete with an applicator hood to ensure your condom gets stuck on and not stuck up. Manufactured by the US company Mentor, and already on sale there, the product is scheduled for launch in the UK later in 1987.

And, for First-Timers

It's time to get the bloody thing on. This is not a question of asking your partner to breathe in, because it won't help at all. And make sure you're not clutching an oriental-sized condom in your hand, unless of course you're bonking an oriental, or there could be real tears before bedtime. Of course, most that follows will also apply if you're gay – in fact, it shouldn't be half as difficult.

Three handy tips:

1. If you have long finger nails we suggest you chew them down before approaching a condom.
2. Always keep a pair of scissors close to the planned site of the act because some of the plastic wrapped condoms are about as inaccessible as Fort Knox. Alternatively you can tear the packaging with your teeth (only recommended if they are your own) in a frenzied passion, but be careful not to sink them into the condom as well.
3. And finally a note for the over-cautious. Do not attempt to blow up your condom before you use it as this will only weaken it. If in doubt, do it afterwards, and then if your worst suspicions are confirmed you still have the morning-after Pill.

Instructions:

The following instructions can only be followed after you have located the piece of anatomy that most closely resembles a skinhead in a polo neck, and it's fully erect (hard, not squidgy).

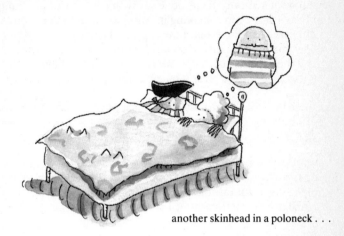

another skinhead in a poloneck . . .

OK, the wrapper is off and you are holding either a rounded or a teat-ended condom in your hand. If you have the latter leave a little extra space at the end of the condom to accommodate the sperm. Different men produce different quantities of sperm, so you may have to weigh him before you start. Making sure the condom is the right way round, hold the teat end between the thumb and fore-finger to expel the air, then roll it down your partner's penis, smoothing out the wrinkles (optional) and avoiding air bubbles. Don't forget to put the condom on before placing the penis into your vagina – it's too narrow inside to put it on afterwards. Now you can have fun.

As soon as it is over, however, remember to remove the penis – *and* the condom. The penis has a tendency to become rather slack and tired after orgasm, not unlike your partner, and then the condom will be too large. At this stage you must avoid all contact with it and its contents because an intrepid sperm may find a way of freeing itself from its latex prison as the penis shrinks, and head straight for the Fallopian tubes. You can ensure your partner doesn't bungle this by holding the penis and condom firmly in your hand and disengaging. Keep an eye on where your partner puts the condom, though – they're twice as lethal as banana skins if you step on one.

A word of caution:

Don't forget to check that neither your partner nor your condom has passed its sell-by date, and remember to use a new one (condom!) every time you do it. And don't try to stretch your supplies out by laundering them, as 12% of those who responded to Journeyman's survey have done. It won't wash out any lingering infections – not even a soaking in 'Bio Tex' will do that – and it will certainly weaken the latex. In exceptional circumstances the law of averages may prove a secondhand Johnny is better than nothing, so for just that special occasion we're including washing instructions taken from a Chinese packet of condoms:

> Wash thoroughly and dust with bathing powder, store in a shaded cool or dry place, preferably in an airtight container to avoid insects and deterioration. Do not use if found stuck together or yellowed.

Remember, don't ever hang your Johnnies on the clothes' line during the day: ultraviolet rays are their greatest enemy. And if you are planning a marathon love-in using the same condom, please disregard all instructions after the word powder.

One last hint:

Many women find that condoms make them sore. This is not the fault of the humble latex Johnny, in most cases it's the fault of the Johnnie who is using it. Men are often far too eager to test the proof worthiness of their raincoats. One way you can prevent your vagina feeling like it has been sandblasted is to use a lubricated condom, or alternatively try a water-based lubricant like 'KY Jelly'. However, don't use 'Vaseline' or any other petroleum-based lubricant because it weakens the latex. The best way to avoid that sandpapered feeling is to treat the cause of the problem and provide your partner with a handy sex manual which includes a generous chapter on foreplay. In extreme circumstances you could contemplate exchanging your partner for a better qualified one! One word of caution when using lubricants, although they help it slip in, it also slips out more easily, causing untold harm to both yourself and your partner!

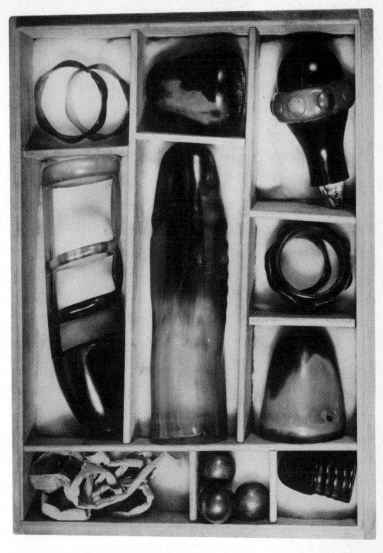

31. A box containing a variety of aids for Japanese love-making, though principally tortoiseshell condoms.

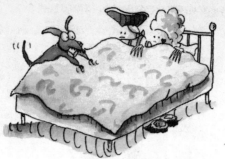

well-trained Yugoslav dogs . . .

Autres pays, autres moeurs
A Rose by any other Name: or

The Cosmopolitan Guide to the Condom

To travel hopefully is better than to arrive, or so we were told in our youth; but what we weren't told is how difficult travelling hopefully can be when you can't communicate with the natives. We all know the story of the Englishman whose wife died when they were on holiday in France. Like all Englishmen, he had naturally got a dark suit with him, but he didn't have a black hat, which he felt he needed to show that he was in mourning. So he decided to buy one in the local department store. Unfortunately, his knowledge of French was a little rusty, so that instead of a 'chapeau noir' (black hat), he asked for 'une capote noire' (a black condom). He was surprised to be sent from the gentlemen's outfitting department to what appeared to be the pharmaceutical section, but felt that this was probably a foreign way of dividing departments that he didn't understand. He repeated his request at the counter, and the assistant asked him why he wanted a black one. 'Because my wife is dead.' 'Ah, Monsieur, quelle délicatesse!' (What refinement).

So that other holiday-makers don't have similar problems, go into shops to buy condoms, and come out with hats, envelopes or gloves, we include here a guide to the usual words for condom in a number of useful languages. We're sorry that not all languages are represented, but we didn't succeed in getting suitable informants for some languages, and many of the experts we wrote to simply didn't reply. Perhaps, gentle readers, we'll be able to fill in these gaps in a later edition – with your help.

We should perhaps point out that phrase books and language

guides hardly ever contain the words for condoms. Why not? God – or the author – only knows. A few years ago *Spare Rib* investigated forty phrase books to see if they had the words for useful things like tampons and condoms – the result? A nil return. Using these phrase books no holiday-maker could buy either tampons or French Letters; yet thirty-eight of them had the word for trapeze! the *Berlitz* guides are now a little better, though even they just have 'contraceptives' and 'sanitary napkins'. They are also quite helpful in the process that might lead up to a visit to the chemist, having a whole section on getting to know people; fortunately it also contains phrases for 'No, I'm not interested' and 'Leave me alone, please'.

Naming of Names

Of course, it is not only a question of language. Brand names must be mentioned, and you'd be surprised just how they vary throughout the world and what they tell you about the indigenous men.

As any marketing person will tell you, to make a product sell you have to give it an appealing name and one that in some way conveys a message that will give you the incentive to buy. This is a question of simple psychology and, of course, the most popular psychological selling ploy is sex. Sex is used to sell everything from cars to chocolates, in fact you can use sex to sell almost anything, as long as it's not really sex. Because as we all know, if we talk about sex and really mean it we're going to offend all those members of the moral majority.

It's therefore no surprise then that the popular brand-named condoms in the UK never reflect how pleasurable sex can be, but skirt around the issue to find more important considerations. Here we extoll the praises of condom safety with names like LRC's '██████' and '██████' mentioned before, or efficiency with flimsy '██████' and delicate '██████' (this should test your knowledge of LRC brand names!). And if reliability and condom thinness are all the average man in this country thinks about when he's having sex, then we're emigrating, but not to Australia, with names like 'Doublecheck' and 'Checkmate' – they're all far too cautious for our liking. We're giving Bangladesh, Jamaica and El Salvador a miss as well. These countries are far too preoccupied with male prowess and supremacy with popular brands called 'Raja (King of Spades)', 'Panther' and 'Condor' (Ah! that condor moment) respectively. And the Americans are just as bad with the 'Trojan' brand (although they obviously associate the word 'Trojan' with strength, rather than the unfortunate fate that befell the Horse). No, we're going to Japan, where they get right down to the nitty gritty, and use brand names that appeal to women and don't mince their words.

Well you can't get more candid than 'Lady Wet' for a brand of
condom can you?

A Word in Your Ear

Although the words are important: where we use the words is
important too. Condoms are sold in a lot of places: slot-machines,
drug stores, department stores, supermarkets, newspaper kiosks,
but obviously not at all these places in every country. The question
of who buys the condoms also differs from country to country. For a
long time, buying condoms was a male preserve. Especially in the
days when the barber's shop was the most popular retail outlet, it
was only the most adventurous women who would have ventured to
buy their own. A lot of less enlightened men found this spirit of
adventure rather disturbing: 'if she buys her own condoms, who can
guarantee that she will only use them with me'? So a basically simple
matter like buying French Letters can lead to jealousy, drama, even
tragedy. But that doesn't apply just to condoms – it's true of all
contraceptives, so we'll pass on quickly. The fact remains that
women have been boldly buying condoms for about twenty years,
even if they've mainly preferred to use self-service chemists, drug
stores and supermarkets.

The siting of sheaths in these self-service outlets tells us a lot
about attitudes to condoms – not on the part of the customers, but of
the management. Some shops display them next to razor blades and
aftershave; thus they expect a male clientele, and by deliberately
putting them in this area, give them a masculine character. Others,
even if it's only a few, put them near sanitary towels and tampons,
which turns the sheaths into an article of 'feminine hygiene'. A lot of
drug stores, particularly in France, put them next to sticking
plasters, which happen to be made by the same firm. In this way the
condom loses its air of mystery or indecency and becomes a simple
household article. The effect of putting condoms and plasters together is charming, since both are intended to deal with little
household accidents: the one before, the other afterwards. On the
other hand, in Stornoway they are put next to disposable nappies,
which doesn't inspire a great deal of confidence.

Since this rich variety of opportunities to purchase condoms
exists, it's amazing that so many people, mostly men, actually
dream of walking the streets without them. Imagine what would
happen if the police in one of the raids they love so much arrested,
not Greenham Common women, hippies or suspected terrorists,
but men who weren't carrying condoms (after all, seat belts are
compulsory now): the prisons would be bursting at the seams before
you could say Johnny. Reliable witnesses (women, of course) who

remember the fifties tell us that in those days no man of the world (DA, drape jacket, drainpipes and crepe soles) would have dreamt of going out without a French Letter. Of course they kept them in their wallets, which as you know is not very good for our little rubber friends. Maybe an enterprising designer will find a way to incorporate them in a 'Filofax'?

Still, we're not concerned with yuppies here, but the simple task of buying condoms. Barbers have been the uncrowned kings among dealers on the international French Letter scene, and traditionally it's been their lot to dispense condoms discreetly to a largely male clientele. Approaching the subject used to take the form of the following: barber brushes hair from back of client's neck and politely inquires, 'a little something for the weekend, sir'. These days Eric and Nick Nicolaou, who have been shaving, snipping and selling condoms from their Old Street barber's shop for twenty years, are far blunter about the subject, merely asking if the client 'wants any French Letters'.

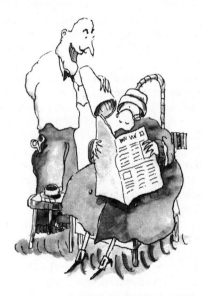

a little something for the weekend, sir . . .

'███████' are the only brand they sell at the moment, both advertising and packets are clearly on view, liberally scattered about the shelves around the shop. Unlike some barbers, Nick and Eric have never kept their condoms secreted beneath the counter; they've always been positioned at eye level, so they're hard to avoid seeing.

Eric claims that no one's ever been remotely embarrassed about asking for them, either. So who are their customers?

> 'Well most of our customers these days are married men, they don't buy '██████' for contraceptive reasons, they buy them to prevent disease, but we've got a lot of female customers as well. I remember years ago we used to sell a brand called 'Paris', and then there were the old fashioned re-usable condoms that we sold for threepence each. We don't sell as many condoms as we used to sell five or six years ago – I don't know why, I think most women take the Pill these days. Our best seller these days is "Stud 100" (a delay action spray to prevent premature ejaculation), we sell more of that stuff than anything else.'

A Buyer's Guide

Britain, or rather English-speaking countries, like the USA and Australia, as well as the English-speaking parts of Wales, Scotland and Ireland. Oh yes, and England too, about which was said – probably by a Mr Shaw: 'People on the Continent have a sex-life. The English use a hot-water bottle'. Was he referring to the quality of condoms at the time?

A lot of the words used have already appeared in earlier chapters, but we might as well recap here. One very common term is the brand name '██████', which like Hoover and Biro has almost become a common noun. From this we get the popular song '██████' is a girl's best friend', and also the occasional whimsical alteration of ICI paint adverts, where the Old English sheepdog exhorts one and all 'You can depend on Dulux' (but don't get them mixed up; there's a limit to the wall area you can cover with a contraceptive, and with the colours they come in nowadays you'll hardly need to paint it).

The most common colloquial term is 'French Letter' – once again the French are credited with great ingenuity in the erotic and sexual field (the Germans, too, call them Parisians), though we should be aware that the French return the compliment, as you will see. The 'Letter' part of the phrase may come from the idea of the condom's enveloping powers; and indeed, the word 'envelope' is also used for the sheath. The 'French' connection may well also live in the term 'frog' and also 'frog-skin', though this may just derive from the clammy feel of the things. Then there's the famous 'Johnny', who so often comes marching home. Why condoms have been christened in this way is not clear, though, Johnny was once a slang term for the penis. This could also be the root of the term 'jo-bag'. Enid Blyton fans will be delighted to hear that she, too, has been active in this field, with the term 'nodder', based on the similarity of the belled cap Noddy wears to the teat condom. We've seen 'glove' in both England and the US, and other kinds of clothing are also pressed into service: 'one-piece overcoat', 'pacamac' (you can always pull one over your head if it's raining), 'diving suit' and the enigmatic and presumably military 'Port Said garters'. Scientifically, as well as condom and sheath, there are the four P's: preventive, preservative, prophylactic, protective.

In the US they are often called 'rubbers': British readers, for whom rubbers are used to erase things rather than prevent them, should beware of going into a stationer's shop in America and asking for them; likewise Americans, even if they do find rubbers in chemists, will probably end up with erasers. '(French) safe' and 'safety' are terms whose meaning is obvious, as is 'skin'.

We've met some military terms before, and 'armour' is another of them, though becoming a little dated. 'Dreadnought' presumably comes both from its literal meaning, and from the battleship, and 'fearnought' seems to have been coined by analogy with this. One wartime term which strikes us as a little worrying is 'Spitfire' – surely spitting is the last thing condoms are supposed to do! 'Trojan' is a trade name, this time American, and is also likely to give rise to anxiety: after all, the Trojan Horse is famed precisely for spilling its contents, which then spread to every corner of the city. And while we're thinking of Freudian symbolism, there is also 'phallic thimble'.

Sloanes, fresh from the Chelsea Flower Show, no doubt, call them 'dibbers', and a lady who misspent her youth at Oxford (one hopes none of her youths misspent) informs us that they were dubbed 'Freds' among the undergrads.

Australia, while using some of the above terms, also provides us with 'lifesaver': advertising from Down Under tells us 'Australia is one of the last outposts of real manhood [and I suppose 'man-hood' could also be a term for condoms], a land where men are men and physical strength is considered a virtue. And the Australian lifesaver embodies, like nobody else, the ideals of Australian manliness . . . Australian lifesavers are the answer to every American woman's prayer'. Why only American women, we hear you cry – but the land of the dingo (which is *not* a sex aid) keeps its secret to itself.

Relatively colourless words like 'gear', 'tackle' and 'thingy' can be used if the context is clear, but then so can '. . . You know . . .' or even '. . .', as in the question 'Have you got a. . .?' Beware however asking for '■■■■' in Australia as it's a well known brand of 'Sellotape' – and you could come seriously unstuck!

Finally, the railways, particularly those massive locomotives that thunder across the American prairies scattering all that stands in their path with the protruberance they carry in front of them, provide us with 'come-catcher'.

Below we have included a selection of the more interesting additional names Journeyman's survey brought to light. Overall, Journeyman found that the usual term was '███████' which accounted for 25%, followed by sheaths (15%), rubbers (12%), French Letters (10%) and condoms (7%). If you know of more, please write to us:

> Dunkies, cum bags, splatter-bags, flunkies, balloons, things, jackets, male items, hats, coso (thingy in Italian!), diving bell, Johnny bags.

And from another source:

> Irish eelskins, baggies, gossies, bishops, joy-bags, and pink soldiers.

As should be obvious by now, all these objects, exotic and not so exotic, can be obtained from chemists, barbers, drug stores and (on the rare occasions they're both there and working) slot-machines.

As sex is not at its best a premeditated act, one would have hoped that slot-machines could be as plentiful as the bubblegum machines they have often been mistaken for ('this chewing gum is awful' as the graffiti goes). Sadly, however, this is not the case. Sex has traditionally been a taboo subject, so the siting of condom sales points has always been as subtle as possible to protect the blushes of the moral majority. Thus it was that the condom didn't even rear its head from under the pharmacists' counter until 1970. Prior to this it was a case of actually mouthing the taboo words in public.

You can stock up free at any of the many NHS family planning clinics and you can buy your condoms at chemists, at some of the more progressive corner shops, or by mail order. You can't pick them up with your weekly shopping unless you shop at one of the few enlightened supermarkets like Asda, who aim to 'supply all things to all people', Tesco, now selling them in a third of their stores, or Safeway. But not in Sainsbury's: 'we're not a chemist'.

Condom buying is limited enough in the broad light of day, but what happens when you want sex at midnight and find yourself empty-handed. Well, if you've got a car you stand a far better chance of tracking down a condom at one of the vending machine outlets in pubs, public conveniences and some petrol stations. You will need, in the majority of cases, to be a man, or a daring woman as most vending machines are situated in strictly male domains.

Although now an accepted part of public convenience furniture, it was not so back in 1969 when a whole spate of interesting news items began to appear in the press. In 1971, students at Wolverhampton Polytechnic decided to stage a sit-in if the Poly's governing council didn't change their minds about allowing contraceptive vending machines on the premises. Wolverhampton, to be fair, were already behind the times condomwise. Leeds University had had one installed since 1969. Their need was obviously greater, though; during the 1967–68 academic year 49 unmarried students had become pregnant. But the most innovative approach to countering what was obviously a serious problem, was a clever scheme hatched by students at Hull University, where a creche with trained baby-minders was to be provided for women with children on campus. And the funds to support the venture? Well, of course, they were to come out of the profits of the University's two vending machines (the machines were at the time dispensing a healthy 432 condoms a week). One does however wonder whether the two things weren't ultimately working against each others' interests.

If you're lucky enough to live anywhere near the King's Road in London you will be able to take advantage of one of the few alfresco dispensing machines in the entire country. Michael Conitzer's 'Jiffi' dispenser is open all hours, and there is no reason why these sorts of dispensers shouldn't be sited everywhere. No law prohibits outside vending machines, apart from a bye-law stating they shouldn't be sited too close to a public highway. Alas, it's that cursed moral majority again assuming that the mere presence of a condom dispenser will turn the average person into a raving sex maniac. Unfortunately the problem is more a question of 'privatisation'. As Michael Conitzer will confirm, the least of his worries is a rapidly emptying condom dispenser – it's the dispenser itself he has to keep replacing.

What follows is a short list of outlets participants in Journeyman's survey would like to see stocking condoms (like the pioneering cafe in Avignon which is now selling them over the counter – with great success, we understand):

> Off-licences, newsagents, women's toilets, restaurants, ice cream vans, petrol stations, clubs and bars, late-night shops (*but most thought everywhere*).

Wales: The English-speaking areas are a hard act to follow, and so Wales has got the sticky end once again. It's strange, anyhow, that a language which in other spheres, particularly the erotic, is so rich and inventive, should have such a limited vocabulary in the French Letter field. But we can only trust our informants.

Some of the Welsh examples are borrowed straight from English: 'Diwrecs', Johnny, Frenchie. Boring. But how about 'sâch dyrnu' (threshing sack)? Then there's 'gêr', probably borrowed from

English 'gear', and wonderful official words which finally show that we are really dealing with Welsh and no other language: 'maneg atal cenhedlu' and 'maneg wrthgenhedlu', which both mean contraceptive glove. There's the word glove again, which we've already found in English, and which we are going to meet many more times during our travels. These things are sold by the chemist (fferyllydd), the barber (eilliwr) or in slot-machines (peiriant slot).

Scotland: Unfortunately we had no Scottish examples until, at the last moment, editorial staff at the *Glasgow Herald* came up with 'bot 'lastic', which roughly translated means elastic member.

Ireland: Here we're talking about the Irish-speaking areas in the Republic (the Gaeltachta), insofar as you can get hold of condoms there at all: we've already mentioned the condom problem in Ireland. Even though French Letters have been legalised, there is still plenty of opposition to them (and other methods of contraception): that can be seen from the very narrow majority of 83 to 80 votes in the Dail when the ban was lifted in April 1985. We don't know whether anyone feels obliged to hand them over in spite of legalisation. We'll leave that to the traveller to find out. We're just assuming that they're available, and giving you the terminology. In the English-speaking areas, by the way, things are no better, but you can use the English words there at least.

First the official terms: 'Frithghiniúint' and 'frithghiniúnach'. Both of these are very general, since the first is a term for all forms of contraception and the second for all contraceptives. But this will get us started; if things get too difficult the chemist can lay out their whole arsenal of devices on the counter for the customer to choose. In Ireland it is really advisable for a man to do the buying. A woman runs the risk of being pestered about her loose living, or to be whisked off into a pub to be converted. Far too many Irishmen feel obliged to prove to the unsuspecting female traveller that a pint o' Harp is a far better pastime that any other: and it doesn't need a condom. In general, people don't talk about it, particularly since some leading figures in the IRA expressed very negative opinions on the question of whether contraceptives should be allowed in the Republic. Nevertheless, the traveller who keeps his or her ear open will hear a few words worth keeping in mind. There is 'craiceann' (skin). The phrase 'bualadh craiceann' (literally beating the skin; actually another word for having it off) shows that condoms are not totally unkown in Irish folk tradition. Similar to this is the word 'leathair' (leather, not letter), and the phrase 'bualadh an leathair'. And then there's 'pilibín', which is rather a sweet word, but is only rarely come across. Originally it meant 'appendage', but has now become a colloquial term for both cock and condom.

The traveller can buy his or her craiceann, leathair or pilibín, as in Wales and England, at the chemist (ceimicí) or the barbers (gruagadóir), but even now, ten of the twelve chemists in Tralee refuse to stock condoms, as do five of the six in Listowel, five of the six in Killarney, not to mention the only one in Cahirciveen. In the absence of slot-machines for French Letters, co-operatives were set up to distribute contraceptives and advice. So you would be well advised before your trip to the Gaeltacht to go to the Sunday flea market in Dublin and stock up from the co-operative stall.

Germany: Very sensibly, Germany doesn't divide into East and West over this matter, because in spite of their other social and political differences, condoms are sold (and used) in the same places on both sides of the Iron Curtain. Since barbers are on the decline as a source, they are left with public loos, drug stores, supermarkets (though there are fewer of those in East Germany) and vending machines. Even the words used are hardly any different: as well as the official 'Kondom' and 'Präservativ' (preservative), the terms 'Pariser' (Parisian) and 'Präser' are in use. Evidence that the French and Gay Paree have connotations of sexual licence among our Teutonic cousins as well. There are a few other terms, found in odd places like Swabia and Hamburg: 'Hemd' (shirt) and 'Nahkampfsocke' (close-combat sock!). As we would expect, most of the rest of Germany shows a very uniform usage, with the exception of Flensburg, where there are no condoms on sale at all, if we are to believe the diary of Heinrich Susemihl: 'Nothing much happens here . . . so you have to spend the whole day drinking beer to console yourself and the nights combing the streets for condom vending machines, which are naturally nowhere to be found.'

France: This means the bits of France where they don't speak Breton, Occitan, Catalan, Basque, Corsican, Alsatian, Flemish or other minority languages. As we already know, French Letters are not called 'lettres francaises' or 'parisiens' in France, but 'capotes anglaises' (English capes or hoods – or car bonnets!). It's interesting how the English and the French both try and leave each other holding the baby in this sort of case, both the positive (well, we think so), like the condom, and the negative, like syphilis, which in France is the 'English' and in England the 'French' disease. This may throw some light on the origin of the terms for condom: since they were first used to prevent infection, they were clearly named after the diseases – a 'French Letter' for a French disease, and an English cape to shelter you from an English one.

English raincoats can be bought in chemists (pharmacie) or in the supermarkets (supermarché, hypermarché), where they are to be found next to 'Nivea' cream, plasters, and cotton wool. Slot-machines are not much in evidence (although they're now being imported from Spain).

Spain: Condoms are sold in the chemist's shop there too. They are called 'perservativo' (preservative) or 'goma hygienica' (hygienic rubber). When we asked about slang terms, our informant told us there weren't any. We were very disappointed, but couldn't get a single syllable out of him.

But he did tell us that French Letters were never forbidden in Spain, even in the darkest days of the Franco regime. The word condom isn't used in Spain, which is a pity, because it has quite a Hispanic ring to it. You could have 'condom' as an abbrevation of 'con condom' (with condom) and 'sindom' for the opposite. Embarraising questions could then be settled very quickly and simply:

Señor (becomes romantic, excited, amoroso, oloroso, etc.)

Señora: 'Condom?'

Señor: 'Sindom'

Señora: 'Cabron!' (a term of abuse, which we are not allowed to translate into English.) On yer bike. Amor's off, dear.

But since that isn't possible, let's pass on to the next country.

Portugal: Chemists sell condoms in Portugal as well, and did so even before the revolution. So Ireland has the somewhat dubious honour of being the only nation in Europe to have persecuted the preventive consistently since its foundation (but even they have seen the error of their ways and are beginning to come round). The word condom doesn't exist in Portuguese either, so that Senhors and Senhoras have missed out on a very informative way of conversing, just like their Spanish cousins. The official term is 'preservativo para homens' (preservative for men). This describes both the condom wearer and the condom buyer, since in Portugal this is also a male preserve. Apart from this, the Portuguese are the only people to have given the condom the beautiful name it deserves: 'camisa de Venus', that is 'Venus' shirt' or 'smock'. Before we get carried away by this mouth-watering word, we should tell you that the phrase is sometimes shortened to the single word 'camisa' (shirt). But that isn't half so romantic, and is used elsewhere (Germany, for example).

Italy: Our Italian informant has given us the official terms first: the politest is 'contraccettivo', but that means any old contraceptive. Then there is 'preservativo' which we probably don't need to translate by now. This is the normal word, which you can happily use in polite company – if you're invited in for coffee with the Doge of Venice, for example. No one will blush, cough or throw you out. In the dictionary you will at long last find the word we missed so sadly in Spanish and Portuguese: 'condom'. But our pleasure was spoilt a little when our informant told us she'd never heard the word used in real life, though someone might once have said 'condoma' in her hearing.

The slang word is – what else? – 'guanto', meaning glove.

You can buy guanti (if you're a man, that is) in chemists, as in so many other countries. There are no sex shops in Italy, we're told, though one is said to have opened recently in Milan, in an inconspicuous corner somewhere. There are obviously no slot-machines either, because of the heat, so the chemist is all that's left.

Cuba: Since the revolution all kinds of contraceptives have been freely available in Cuba. Condoms (the words are the same as in Spanish) are available in every chemist, but so far they're not used much. 'Bloody machismo' (heavy sighs from Cuban women) is to blame, which doesn't just turn down condoms, though, but all other contraceptives as well, because in its book a real man has to produce as many children as possible. A female pioneer of the condom movement in Cuba informs us that her first article on the topic caused a scandal. Simply the use of the word 'condom' (at least the word is in use there) was like a red rag to the sensibilities of the Cuban bulls; that a woman should write about such offensive things was the last straw. She didn't give up, though, and at Christmas she sent them gift-wrapped to a number of young doctors. One of them was insulted at first, but then acquired the taste and sent one back inscribed with greetings. He kept the rest. People who obstinately refused to use them were told they were aphrodisacs, and that helped; as did the fact that a lot of Cubans suffer from gonorrhoea (how things repeat themselves!). Another problem is the poor supply of condoms. Until recently they were imported from China; they 'rot after a while, they have no lubrication, they're far too short. It's obviously a pain to use things like this. And they're not very safe, because they've often become porous after being stored for so long. We use condoms mainly as balloons for children's parties.'

Fortunately, they're now importing condoms from other countries, and they are enjoying an increase in popularity among Cubans of both sexes. So if you're travelling to Cuba, you don't need to take 40,000 with you, you can get what you need in the chemist.

Norway: The official term is 'kondom' (and not 'kordon' as some people erroneously believe). But this latter still exists in the popular word 'kardong'. Kardong is shortened to 'dong', and there we have the term that is the equivalent of French Letter. (There is no knowing whether they have luminous protruberances.) You can

buy dongs in chemists and drug stores, which are often self-service.
If there's no chemist about, barbers or slot-machines will do. Slot-
machines are usually to be found on stations or near public conveniences, but not in pubs.

Sweden: In Sweden things are the same as in Norway, both as
regards language and availability. But we must specially emphasise
the fact that in Sweden there are outsize (XL) condoms for the
extra-well-endowed. It would probably be useful to have extra
small condoms for little people, which might prevent many an
accident caused by a condom slipping off, but there is as much
likelihood that today's men would buy them as their grandfathers
would buy tip condoms. Bloody machismo!

Wherever they are on sale, you'll find reference to 'P-moijligheter'
(P-possibilities: P for preservative) which are advertised in every
village and every hotel. New visitors are confused by this, but old
Sweden hands can make use of the facility and take home some
extra large goodies for their nearest and dearest.

The Netherlands: Even in the land of the Dutch cap, condoms are
on sale – in chemists and supermarkets. (This is getting a little
boring, and it if were not for Yugoslavia, we'd be close to despair.)
And they're called 'kondom', often altered to the friendly nickname
'het kondoomtje'. Then we have the word 'kapotje', which means
nothing else but our friend (not hood or cape or anything similar),
an international word which leads to real *entente cordial*, the
French, Dutch and Turks all joining hands over a condom. Talking
about hands, we mustn't fail to tell you that a Dutch encyclopedia
defines condoms – no, not as gloves, but as 'rubber finger-stalls'. If
they didn't at the same time tell you what part of the body they're
supposed to be worn on, we'd have serious doubts about Dutch
methods of contraception.

Iceland: Firstly, they have the word 'verjur' (protection), which is
the official description. Just as socially acceptable is 'smokkar'
(which originally meant those things that clerks used to put on to
save their cuffs from getting inky). You need to be a little more
careful with 'stigfel' (boot) and 'klofbussur' (hiking boot). Cuff
covers and walking boots are sold in the chemist (lifjabud) and the
gents. In the gents they're sold in slot-machines, not by special
condom salesmen.

To buy them at the chemist, you say: 'ég aetla ad fǎ verjur' (I'd
like some protection). The chemist (it's usually a woman) will then
ask you which brand. If she gets no answer, she'll open a drawer and
show you a selection of her wares. The customer should then point
to the sort required (preferably with the hand).

In the Second World War French Letters were hard to come by in Iceland, and they were also thicker than the modern kind, so people often used them several times, after washing them, of course. One Sunday in a little fishing village in South Iceland a French Letter was hanging on the line to dry. The man next door, Magnus (perhaps a relative of our own mastermind) noticed this. He felt like a little dalliance himself, so he knocked on the door. When the neighbour opened it, Magnus asked if he could borrow the condom for a short time. But the neighbour shook his head regretfully and said: 'Sorry, Magnus, I can't lend you the sheath. It's not mine: it belongs to the male voice choir.'

Yugoslavia: But only the bits that speak Serbo-Croat. There the word is 'persativ'. The origin of the word is clear, and it seems likely that it comes from official usage rather than slang. Our informant couldn't tell us of any other terms. In Yugoslavia persativs are sold, not in chemists and drug stores, nor in flea markets, but in newspaper kiosks. How practical. Every morning you could collect your condom along with your daily paper. They say that it isn't the custom in Yugoslavia to train dogs to fetch condoms – but why not, since they can already bring the papers. Perhaps Yugoslav pet-owners are afraid that their furry friends' canines might pierce the fine skin of their persativs.

Soviet Union: But only the Russian-speaking parts, and even there we're a little in the dark. It's hard enough to understand the Russian soul, as Tolstoy could have told you: there's no way of getting at the Red condom. So all we know is that our little friend is called 'gandón' in Russia. But whether rushing across Red Square shouting 'Gandón' at the top of your voice would get you what you want, we hardly dare to guess. What does this mysterious word from the land of vodka and the balalaika mean in our more prosaic language? Who can guess? Why, glove, of course.

Turkey: Where are French Letters sold in Turkey? In the bazaar? Alas no, the answer is far more down to earth. Even under the green crescent there are chemists and barbers, and the traveller (here, too, the male traveller is advised to take this job over from his female fellow-traveller) can get what he wants by using the magic word – which is 'kaputt'. To anyone who knows any German, this might seem a little alarming, since kaputt is the last thing you'd want them to be; but the word is actually borrowed from the French, and once again means 'car-bonnet' or 'gas-cape'.

And there we must end our international guide to condoms for the moment.

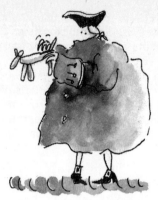

French Letter art . . .

Condom Curiosities

Since we have mentioned many of the most well-known condoms, we are ending our book with a selection of unusual, unknown and even misunderstood condoms. It will not exhaust the theme by any means, but if this book brings you a new awareness, you will recognise that we live in a Mondo Condom, where French Letters are to be found, either in reality or symbolically, at the centre of life, the universe and everything.

Hi-tech Condoms

A revolutionary new idea has been developed in Sweden. It is an aerosol spray, which looks just like any other aerosol, and bears the following label:

> Protective plastic skin, for use against dirt, rust and damp. Prevents short-circuits in the electrical system.

This new wonder spray is sold in garages all over Sweden. It can be sprayed straight onto the penis, and prevents it from short-circuiting. This must be comforting news for men everywhere. It also prevents dirt, rust and damp – everything the old ones were useful for. However, there is a catch, no way has yet been found to remove it, so unless you are into cheese-graters we wouldn't advise using it.

The Condom-Suit

It's true: that's what the Scandinavians (and Clive James in his reviews of Ski Sunday) call those very tight-fitting plastic suits that skiers wear. But these very practical articles of clothing aren't just useful for skiing: they are ideal for everyone who wants to be permanently safe, whether in order to avoid conception, or herpes on any part of the body.

Condom suits are made of nylon or something similar, and ensure that there is a place for everything and that everything is in its place. They can be supplied with or without hood. Ski-racers, batmen (and sometimes supermen, who have the strange habit of wearing their Y-fronts outside the condom-suit) prefer the sort with a hood. The more reckless ski-jumpers prefer the hoodless variety, but then tend to wear helmets.

French Letter Art

Renate Bertlmann is a Viennese artist who has devoted herself to the themes of eroticism and asceticism. She has been working in French Letters for some time, and the things she can do with our flexible friends are quite amazing – if you're interested, see her catalogue 'Discorso "Erotic und Askese" 1984'.

Condom Town

A day in Condom is quite a feat if you can manage it without the damned thing slipping off. But to be serious: you also need to avoid Mondays and Bank Holidays, more particularly Bank Holiday Mondays, otherwise, like our research team, you may end up with less than perfect results: 'We went to Condom, and it was shut!'

Condom is a sleepy little place of just under 4,000 inhabitants in the Department of Gers, and lies on the River Baïse. You need to be careful of the dots on the ï, otherwise the word is pronounced differently, and means something obscene – though possibly quite suitable for the activity that takes place in condoms, if not in Condom itself. It prides itself on its cathedral, and on its position as the centre of the Armagnac industry. Condom en Armagnac – sounds a little chewy as flavour of the month, and if taken too literally could, while perhaps having antiseptic qualities, also sting a little – and too much friction might lead to flambé'd genitalia.

A walk around Condom produced a lot of interesting information: firstly the fact that on a Bank Holiday it's very difficult to get hold of a condom in Condom! The chemists were all closed, and the supermarkets seemed (in spite of what we say elsewhere) not to stock the things. Only when we were driving away in despair at the end of the day did we come across a hypermarket (aptly named Intermarché) at the edge of town where, lo and behold, twelve-packs were available: evidently the inhabitants don't use them often, but when they do, they really go for it.

The Grammatical Condom

You should be well aware by now that the mediaeval Irish, unlike their modern descendants, were enthusiastic users of condoms. If you don't believe it, here's an extract from Thurneysen's Old Irish Grammar:

co n-accae		intí do-eim[1]
(so that) he saw.		he who prot
me	condom accae	do-dot-eim
thee	condot accae	do-dot-eim
him	con(d)id n-accae	do-dn-eim
her	conda accae	do-da-eim
it	con(d)id accae	do-d-eim
us	condon accae	do-don-eim
you	condob accae	do-dob-eim
them	conda accae	do-da-eim
	in tan ro-n-ánaic,	intí nád chúala
	when he reached.	he who has not heard
me	ro-n-dom-ánaic[2]	náchim chúala
thee	ro-n-dot-ánaic	náchit chúalae
him	ro-n-dn-ánaic	nách cúalae
her	ron-da-ánaic	nácha cúalae
it	ro-n-d-ánaic	náchid chúalae
us	ro-n-don-ánaic	náchin cúalae
you	ro-n-dob-ánaic	náchib cúalae
them	ro-n-da-ánaic	nácha cúalae

1 or sg. i do-m-eim
2 do-t-eim; pl.
1 do-n-eim
2 do-t (Class A)
1 or sg. i ro-m-ánaic
2 ro-t-ánaic; pl. ro-n-i-ro-b-ánaic (Class A).

The Condominium

A lot of young Americans now live in condominiums: it is very pleasing to think that they are so responsible and sensible that they ensure birth control by their very way of living. Another kind of condominium is the kind that Britain and France had in the Cameroons when they took them over from Germany after the First World War – probably in the hope of growing rubber trees to supply the ever-growing need for latex. As a legal term condominium means something that is owned in common by several people – like an Icelandic French Letter belonging to a choir.

French Polishing

This is obviously the term for the final step in the process of making *baudruches superfines*.

Military Condoms

In October 1985, 541,000 condoms were ordered by the Australian Ministry of Defence. They were to be used by the Army to protect the mouths of its guns from rusting, including those on tanks. Condoms allow the soldiers to use their guns without having to remove them. It seems they do not deflect bullets, as conventional protection does. The Australian Energy Secretary, Gareth Evans, said that this method is not to be found in any military handbook, but is reliable nonetheless.

Family Condoms

At the 1986 Berlin Film Festival a short film by our American cousin, Dean Parisot, was widely acclaimed to be one of the best of that year's crop. Its title is 'Tom goes to the bar' and during twelve minutes shows Tom's desperate attempts to extract condoms from a slot-machine which stubbornly refuses to accept his coins.

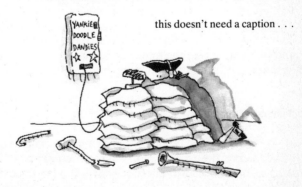

this doesn't need a caption . . .

Condo the Clown

No one could have guessed that an executive director of the Western Australian Family Planning Association would wake up one day to find that he had changed into a giant condom, destined to expose himself in public places for the next three years. But, ridiculed and scorned, Condo the Clown has at last been accepted – even by his own children. He has had such an effect on Western Australians that a national survey has found that they now prefer condoms more than any other Australian. Condo hopes that his Mini-Moke will change into a Condomobile this year and give him a chance to joy-ride rather than parade the streets under a hot sun.

Still, luckily for him he doesn't live in Queensland, where the Prime Minister Sir John Bjelke-Petersen backs the statewide banning of condom vending machines on the pretext they promote promiscuity. The mind boggles at what he would do to a giant condom from Western Australia.

Sea Condoms

It appears that condoms are also a useful aid in efforts to keep beaches cleaner. No, they do not trawl the coastline at night clearing pollution, but as David Bellamy, the well-known botanist explained, the sea shore condom count provides a fairly good measure of the efficiency of a coastal town's sewage disposal. Actually we prefer the trawler condom explanation!

No Love on the Dole

Herr Franz Schmidt of Bremen was most disgruntled after the failure of his appeal to a local social security tribunal. In Germany, unemployment payments are based on the cost of a 'shopping basket' of necessities, and Herr Schmidt argued that condoms should be included (as are cinema tickets). Not so, said the tribunal, presumably feeling that the minds of the unemployed should be on higher things – or providing offspring for the state.

After-Dinner Condoms

If you go out to dinner in Odense in Denmark, be on your guard when they serve the coffee. Don't slip the contents of that little packet into your mouth without checking first: at least one restaurant there is contributing to the 'safe sex' campaign by handing out condoms rather than after-dinner mints, ensuring that any post-prandial canoodling won't have unforeseen results.

Recession Dressing

Price and embarrassment has always hindered young teenagers obtaining condoms, but this added to the Victoria Gillick campaign, when under-16s were even more inhibited about getting supplies, resulted in the emergence of a new phenomenon, namely cling film contraception. Of course a pound's worth of that wrapped around a penis will go a long way, but unfortunately not very far in preventing pregnancy. We've also heard of a case where a crisp packet was employed, but what flavour, brand, size or indeed consequences are unknown. If it was you, dear reader, please let us know, we're speechless.

Plastic Condoms

No, these are not to be found near holes on motorways, but it seems that the Americans did attempt to make plastic condoms during the last war. Apparently their efforts came to nothing because of the high insulating qualities of plastic compared to latex. Maybe the US space industry should turn its attention to this little problem – well, they came up with non-stick frying pans, didn't they?

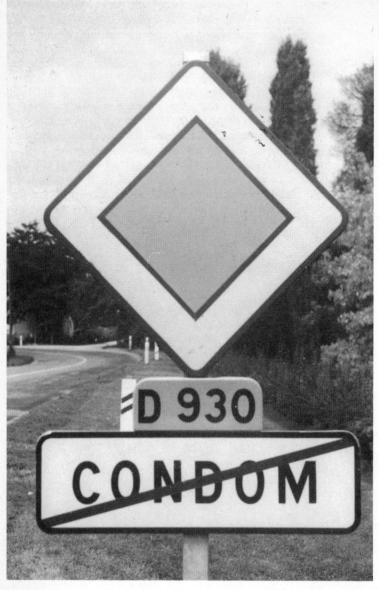

32. Horror-struck you should be – YOU ARE NOW LEAVING CONDOM!

Dear readers,

While reading our book you probably remembered many other condom-facts, stories or references about our friend in literature, as well as more names it is called across the world. Please let us know, and if we publish them in our next edition, we will send you a free copy.

And remember, especially our male readers, *you should always have it on before you have it off!*

Appendix: Survey

What follows is a brief summary of the results arising out of a survey undertaken by Journeyman during September 1986, some of which have already been referred to in the body of the text.

With the assistance of three suppliers, seven condoms were sent to individuals who had responded to editorial coverage of the survey in CITY LIMITS, TIME OUT, NEW SOCIETY, FORUM and CAPITAL GAY.

The aim of the survey was to ask some general questions, and undertake tests on several varieties of condoms: two very standard ones (specifically purchased for the survey because LRC Products refused to help); and delayed-reaction, ribbed, coloured, flavoured and teatless versions.

Over 250 questionnaires and samples were sent to participants scattered around the country, and 82 were returned completed, involving 159 people. 68 principal respondents were men (out of which 9 were gay) and 14 were women.

The conclusions we drew from this exercise were that although we fully recognised the unscientific nature of the questionnaire and sample, it was clear that more research should be undertaken, especially now that the condom has once again proved its effectiveness as a barrier against infection, as well as a contraceptive.

As far as we know, most surveys on condoms are closely linked to market research and are not available for public use. Social attitudes are likely to change quite quickly as a result of AIDS, and possibly even faster than the arbiters of what we are allowed to see and hear. If the sole manufacturer of condoms in this country still sees the market as "conservative", it will respond conservatively, whether or not large sections of that market have changed. The result has been the marginalisation of the condom, and the success of alternative means of contraception like the Pill. Fortunately for the condom industry, the Government is spending £20 million to try and reverse this trend, but it will need the imagination of the Swedish advertising campaigns of the seventies to build on any short-term gains.

So, back to the survey: the questionnaire is reproduced over the next four pages. Following that is a breakdown of the answers to questions 6 to 16, according to whether they were completed by a MALE-FEMALE partner; MALE-MALE partner; FEMALE-MALE partner. A general point first, though: the majority of male respondents were aged between 25 and 34 (4 were over 65); and were in full-time work, primarily in the service industry and education. The largest number of gays were aged between 45 and 54. Most of the women respondents were aged between 16 and 24, and were still in full-time education.

116

THE JOURNEYMAN CONDOM SURVEY

September 1986

We have sent you this questionnaire because we would like to know what you and your partner(s) think of condoms – and in particular the free samples enclosed! <u>YOUR REPLIES WILL BE TREATED IN STRICT CONFIDENCE</u>.

Please answer the questions and return the completed form to the address below by 30 September. All those received by that date will be entitled to a 25% discount off the retail price of <u>JOHNNY COME LATELY: A Short History of the French Letter</u> by Jeannette Parisot. This fascinating new book will be published in November by Journeyman at £4.95, and will include the analysed results of the survey. It will also contain vouchers providing discounts for additional quantities of the condoms you tested, and many more varieties!

To maintain anonymity, please complete the address slip and return it to us, either with your questionnaire or separately, by the end of September. By way of confirmation of its receipt we will send you a <u>FREE</u> copy of a "censored" edition of one of our earlier books!

First some general questions, which can be completed even if you are not a regular user of condoms. Most are designed to be ticked off, but where you think a longer answer is required, please elaborate.

1. Are you male or female?   Male ☐01   Female ☐02

2. What is your partner's sex? Male ☐01   Female ☐02

3. What is your age?

under 16 ☐01   16 – 24 ☐02   25 – 34 ☐03   35 – 44 ☐04

  45 – 54 ☐05   55 – 64 ☐06   65 or over ☐07

4. What is your working status?

Full time ☐01   Part time ☐02   Unemployed ☐03

Student ☐04   School student ☐05

5. What is your occupation?

Service industry ☐01   Manual ☐02   Education ☐03

Administration ☐04

Other, please specify:...

6. What do you think is the greatest benefit condoms offer?

Protection against sexually-transmitted diseases ☐01

As a contraceptive, without side effects ☐02

Both equally as important ☐03

7. If you use condoms for contraception, is it your usual method?

Yes ☐01   No ☐02

(a) If NO, what do you or your partner normally use?

Pill ☐01   Coil ☐02   Pessaries ☐03   Foam ☐04

Jelly ☐05   Rhythm method ☐06

Other, please specify:..

(b) If YES, do you or your partner use additional protection?

Yes ☐01   No ☐02

If you do, please specify:...

8. How effective a form of birth control do you think condoms are?

Very effective ☐01   Effective enough for most people's needs ☐02

One of the less effective methods ☐03

9. Which of the following most accurately describes your feelings about using a condom?

Condoms introduce some variety into sex ☐01

Condoms take the spontaneity out of sex ☐02

Condoms make sex more fun ☐03

Condoms make sex seem clumsy and fumbly ☐04

10. When you purchase condoms, which of these suppliers do you normally use?

Chemist ☐01   Family-planning clinic ☐02   Hairdresser ☐03

Vending machine ☐04   Mail order ☐05   Supermarket ☐06

Other, please specify:..

11. Do you find condoms embarrassing to purchase? Yes ☐01 No ☐02

12. Where else would you prefer to purchase condoms? For example, in off-licences, or newsagents?

Please specify:...

13. Do you ever re-use condoms?   Yes ☐01   No ☐02

14. What do you generally call condoms?

Please specify:...

15. Do you think condoms should be advertised on radio and television?

Yes ☐01   No ☐02

16. Do you think condoms should be more easily available to the under-16s?

Yes ☐01   No ☐02

And now to the practical aspects of our survey!

<u>HAVE A GOOD TIME!</u>

17. We have sent you seven different condoms to test. Please rate each one on the characteristics listed below. We would also like to have your partner's opinions - although we recognise that not all of the questions will be applicable!

Just place the number which reflects your views in each box:

1 Very Good 2 Good 3 Average 4 Fair 5 Poor

		Ease of unwrapping 01	Ease of fitting 02	Size 03	Appearance 04	Sensitivity 05	Prolongs intercourse 06	Shortens intercourse 07
PARTNER	Prophyltex Red Stripe							
	D---x F------e							
	D---x G-----r							
	Jiffi Prolong							
	Jiffi Ribbed							
	Aegis Coloured							
	Aegis Fruity							
YOURSELF	Prophyltex Red Stripe							
	D---x F------e							
	D---x G----r							
	Jiffi Prolong							
	Jiffi Ribbed							
	Aegis Coloured							
	Aegis Fruity							

* Note: Because a selection of "coloured" and "fruity" condoms are being tested, please specify which colour or aroma you received:

Fruity.......................... Coloured.............................

Journeyman would like to express its thanks to the newspapers and magazines which carried our request for participants, and to the suppliers for the free samples - excluding the London Rubber Company, manufacturers of D---x condoms, who refused to co-operate.

18. This question only requires the description which is closest to you and your partner's opinion to be ticked off. Hopefully it will not be too arduous, and may even give "rise" to some fun!

LUBRICATION			TEXTURE			TASTE			SMELL			COLOUR				
Dry	Perfect	Oily	Stimulating	Ineffective	Uncomfortable	Enjoyable	Tasteless	Nasty	Attractive	Rubbery	Unpleasant	Exciting	Colourless	Revolting		
															Aegis Fruity	YOURSELF
															Aegis Coloured	
															Jiffi Ribbed	
															Jiffi Prolong	
															D---x G----r	
															D---x F----e	
															Prophyltex Red Stripe	
															Aegis Fruity	PARTNER
															Aegis Coloured	
															Jiffi Ribbed	
															Jiffi Prolong	
															D---x G----r	
															D---x F----e	
															Prophyltex Red Stripe	
15	14	13	12	11	10	09	08	07	06	05	04	03	02	01		

Thank you for taking the trouble to complete the questionnaire. We expect that the analysed results will provoke a great deal of interest when <u>JOHNNY COME LATELY</u> is published, so don't miss out on our special prepublication offer!

QUESTION	MALE-FEMALE (%)	MALE-MALE (%)	FEMALE-MALE (%)
6. Are condoms best as:			
protection against STDs	13	44	7
contraceptive	18	0	21
both equally	68	56	71
7. Are condoms usual method	50	33	64
7a. If no: normally Pill	46	0	100
7b. If yes: do use			
additional protection: yes	17	0	22
no additional protection	86	33	78
8. As a contraceptive:			
Very effective	37	22	29
Effective enough	54	33	50
Not effective	3	11	21
9. Condoms:			
introduce variety	35	44	21
reduce spontaneity	21	22	43
make sex more fun	12	11	21
make sex clumsy	16	11	7
10. Which normal suppliers:			
chemist	43	44	64
family-planning clinic	7	0	14
hairdresser	1	0	0
vending machine	7	11	0
mail order	12	0	7
supermarket	7	11	7
11. Embarrassing to buy:			
yes	31	22	36
no	68	78	64
13. Do you ever re-use them:			
yes	12	22	14
no	88	78	86
15. Should they be advertised:			
yes	72	89	71
no	28	11	29
16. Should they be easily available to the under-16s:			
yes	79	67	93
no	19	33	7

The second set of figures provides a breakdown of answers to questions 7, 9, 15 and 16; followed by a graphical representation of answers to questions 7, 15 and 16 from the largest sample (all males).

QUESTIONS by age (%)	16-24 M	F	25-34 M	F	35-44 M	F	45-54 M	F	55-64 M	F	64+ M	F	all M/F
7. Usual method	44	63	57	50	57	100	54	–	40	–	50	–	57
9. Adds variety	22	25	39	25	50	0	15	–	20	–	75	–	30
lacks spontaneity	33	38	17	50	29	50	23	–	0	–	0	–	27
makes more fun	0	25	13	0	7	50	15	–	20	–	25	–	17
makes sex clumsy	22	0	13	25	14	0	23	–	20	–	0	–	13
15. Yes to TV advertising	78	75	74	75	93	50	62	–	60	–	25	–	66
16. Yes for under-16s	89	88	78	100	100	100	62	–	60	–	75	–	84

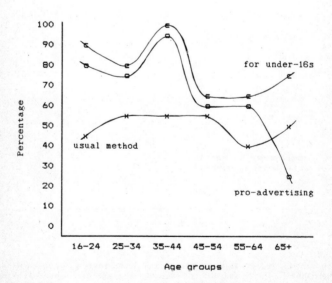

Some conclusions, by question:

6. Clearly the majority of participants felt that condoms were equally important as both a protection and as a contraceptive, although a higher proportion of gays saw protection as more important.

7. Because of the type of questionnaire it was, a high percentage of participants use condoms as their principal form of contraception — especially in the 25 to 44 year age group. Of those who don't, the Pill is the most common (small percentages used the other methods of contraception listed — generally no more than 5% — and the following: Dutch cap, vasectomy/sterilisation, withdrawal and a bottle of scotch). Over 75% of those who use condoms do not use any other form of protection (those who do, use spermicidal jellies and pessaries).

8. Generally everyone thought that the condom was effective enough for most people's needs, although a higher percentage of women didn't think it was effective enough.

9. In the main, men seemed to feel that condoms brought some variety to sex; although women felt that it took the spontaneity out of sex, condoms could make it more fun.

10. The vast majority of both men and women purchase their condoms from the chemist, but women also use the family-planning clinics.

11. Two-thirds no longer find it embarrassing to buy condoms.

13. Interestingly, one person in ten has re-used their condoms.

15. The majority of participants thought condoms should be advertised, in particular more gays than heterosexuals, and especially in the 35 to 44 year age group.

16. A slightly larger majority (except gays) thought that condoms should be more easily accessible to the under-16s, especially the women.

With the questionnaire, each participant was sent seven condoms about which several questions were asked concerning colour, smell, taste, texture and lubrication; and more specific questions about individual qualities.

First the more general questions:

COLOUR

The majority (67%) considered all were colourless, except Aegis Fruity and Coloured — over half thought these exciting, and a third revolting. Unfortunately many could not make up their minds which smell they had: 74% thought strawberry, 9% raspberry, 6% cherry and 11% were unsure.

SMELL

The majority considered all smelt rubbery, except Aegis Fruity — 62% thought these were attractive and 25% unpleasant. (Also 23% thought Aegis Coloured had an attractive smell.)

TASTE

Nearly all thought the condoms tasted nasty, or were tasteless. Only Aegis Fruity was thought enjoyable (64%), but 25% thought it nasty.

TEXTURE

Over half thought textures were ineffective, but half considered Jiffi Ribbed and Red Stripe stimulating (and a third ineffective).

LUBRICATION

Over half considered lubrication perfect, but almost a third thought Aegis Fruity , Coloured and Aegis Delay oily (a high proportion of Jiffi Prolongs were substituted with Aegis Delay); Jiffi Ribbed and Red Stripe were thought dry.

OVERALL: Best on average was Aegis Fruity, which seemed to be liked because of its colour, smell and taste. Worst was "D---x" G------r and Aegis Delay, both of which were considered colourless, rubbery and tasteless to nasty. The others scored on a few points, but not enough to make them exceptionally good or bad.

And now for the specific questions:

EASE OF UNWRAPPING

Easiest were Red Stripe, "D---x" F--------e and G------r, and Aegis Coloured.

EASE OF FITTING

All average to good, Jiffi Ribbed slightly less so.

SIZE

Best was "D---x" F--------e, worst Jiffi Ribbed, but all average.

APPEARANCE

Majority average, but best was Red Stripe (17% above average)

SENSITIVITY

Definitely best was "D---x" F--------e, followed by Red Stripe and Jiffi Ribbed. Rest average.

PROLONGS INTERCOURSE

Only Aegis Delay had any effect (21% above average).

SHORTENS INTERCOURSE

All average (except of course the above), with "D---x" F--------e slightly better.

OVERALL: Averaging the statistics over ease of unwrapping, fitting, size, appearance and sensitivity: "D---x" F--------e and Red Stripe are rather better than average (20% and 19%); next best "D---x" G------r and Aegis Coloured (13% and 10%); with Aegis Delay, Jiffi Ribbed and Aegis Fruity close to average (6%, 7% and 9%).

In running order: on general questions, the best is "D---x"
F--------e and Red Stripe, followed by "D---x" G------r, Aegis
Coloured, Aegis Fruity, Jiffi Ribbed, Aegis Delay.
On specific qualities, the best was Aegis Fruity, Aegis Coloured, Red
Stripe, "D---x" F--------e, Jiffi Ribbed, Aegis Delay, "D---x"
G------r.

COMMENTS FROM THE PARTICIPANTS

"Black is the only colour that turns me on"

"Condoms are much more fun when fitted on by the partner"

"The smell is also exciting as it promises things to come"

"Condoms are no problem once you get used to them; at the beginning I
couldn't keep my erection"

"We did not like vivid colours"

"My partner found Red Stripe uncomfortable after ejaculation because
there is no nipple"

"Godamawful 'Burning Rubber tyre' smell"

Journeyman Help *Directory*

The following addresses and telephone numbers can be used to obtain advice and information; any contact will be treated in the strictest confidence. Otherwise the best place to go for help is your own GP (who cannot prescribe condoms).

CONTRACEPTION AND FAMILY PLANNING

NHS family planning clinics: see local telephone directory under Family Planning Services. Free information on all methods of birth control, and free supplies on prescription.

The Family Planning Association, 27–35 Mortimer Street, London W1N 7RJ. (01) 636 7866. Free leaflets on methods and information about family planning services. The FPA also have regional offices in Bedford, Belfast, Birmingham, Brighton, Cardiff, Exeter, Glasgow, Liverpool, Norwich and Sheffield.

FPA Book Centre, at above London address. Books on contraception and sexuality: free book list.

Family Planning Sales Ltd, 28 Kelburne Road, Cowley, Oxford, OX4 3SZ. FPA mail-order contraceptives.

Brook Advisory Centres for Young People, Central Office, 153a East Street, London, SE17 2SD. (01) 708 1234. Free birth control advice and supplies for young people. Regional centres in Birmingham, Bristol, Burnley, Coventry, Edinburgh, Liverpool.

Family Planning Clinic, Marie Stopes House, The Well Woman Centre, 108 Whitfield Street, London W1. (01) 388 0662. Free birth control advice and information. Regional vasectomy and sterilisation centres can be contacted through London.

Women's Global Network on Reproductive Rights, PO Box 4098, Minahassastraat 1, 1009 AB Amsterdam, Netherlands. (020) 923900. Autonomous network open to all individuals and groups who support reproductive rights for women.

Women's Reproductive Rights Information Centre, 52 Featherstone Street, London EC1. (01) 251 6332.

SEXUALLY TRANSMITTED DISEASES AND AIDS

NHS sexually transmitted diseases clinics, Special Clinics or GU (genito-urinary) clinics: see local telephone directory under Venereal Disease, or your nearest main hospital. Free advice and help in the strictest confidence.

Terrence Higgins Trust, BM/AIDS, London WC1N 3XX. Helpline (01) 833 2971. Help and counselling to infected persons: offers detailed information on safe sex.

London Lesbian and Gay Switchboard, BM Switchboard, WC1 3XX. (01) 837 7324. Answers general enquiries about AIDS; has directory of local gay support groups and STD clinics.

Body Positive, contacted through Trust Helpline or Lesbian and Gay Switchboard above from 7 – 10 pm each day. Self-help group of gay men.

Health Education Council, 73 New Oxford Street, London, WC1. (01) 637 1881. For single free copies of *AIDS — what everybody needs to know*, write to Dept A, PO Box 100, Milton Keynes, MK1 1TX.

Healthline Telephone Service, (01) 981 2717, (01) 980 7222 (outside London, 0345 581151 to be charged at local rate). Up-to-date 24-hour recorded information on AIDS and advice on safe sex.

Welsh AIDS Campaign, c/o HEACW, Secretariat, Room 2003, Welsh Office, Cathays Park, Cardiff, CF1 3NQ. (0222 823395).

Scottish AIDS Monitor, PO Box 169, Edinburgh (031) 558 1167.

DHSS AIDS Unit, Alexander Fleming House, Elephant and Castle, London, SE1 6BY. (01) 403 1893.

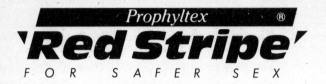

Prophyltex ®
'Red Stripe'
F O R   S A F E R   S E X

The 'Red Stripe' Collection

———

To receive by return:

1. A 6 pack of 'Red Stripe'
   the long strong teatless condom

2. An XL American cut Red Stripe
   (Tell Willie) grey cotton T Shirt

3. A Red Stripe gas lighter

Simply send a cheque or P.O. (no cash please) for £7.50 (plus 25p P&P)
to F.T.C.
2 Ladbroke Grove London W11

There is no need to remove this page to order 'Red Stripe', as a letter stating you have seen this ad will suffice

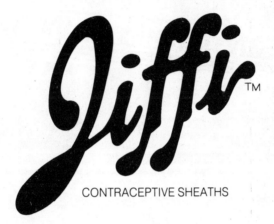

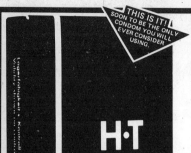
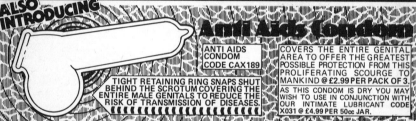
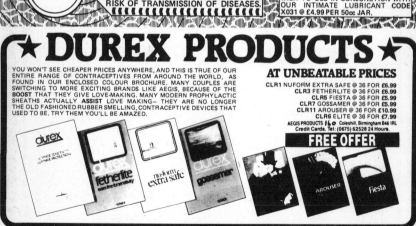